Medical Errors
and Adverse Events:
Managing the Aftermath

Medical Errors
and Adverse Events:
Managing the Aftermath

David Waluube

ISBN: Hardcover   978-1-4653-5401-3
               Softcover   978-1-4628-4658-0
               Ebook   978-1-4653-5400-6

This book was printed in the United States of America.

To order additional copies of this book, contact:
Xlibris Corporation
0-800-644-6988
www.xlibrispublishing.co.uk
Orders@xlibrispublishing.co.uk
302125

CONTENTS

Dedicated to *Mary,* my mother, *Mary,* my wife, my *children,* and grandchildren.

Preface

In health care, the rising complexities and reach of modern medicine have produced startling levels of risk and harm to patients. Serious or potentially serious medication errors occurred in 6.7 per cent of patients in one study in two highly regarded hospitals in the world, admittedly, many years ago now. The Harvard Medical Practice Study of 1984, which reviewed 30,000 hospital records in New York State, USA, found injuries from medical care to occur in 3.7 per cent of hospital admissions. Over 50 per cent of these injuries were preventable and 13.6 per cent of these were fatal. The cost of medical errors is high, both in financial, social, and professional terms. Statistics like these have influenced the ongoing mobilisation of public and professional sentiments to redesign health care products and devices, improve on faulty systems, and make health products and devices much safer.

When medical errors and adverse events occur, the reaction in medical settings is most commonly an attempt to fix blame and to punish someone. This, usually, is counterproductive. Fear, reprisal, and punishment produce not safety, but rather defensiveness, secrecy, and enormous human anguish. In complex systems, safety depends not on exhortation, but rather on the proper design of equipments, job planning, support systems, and organisations. Safer care systems do produce safer care.

In the USA, effective safety improvements have happened since the formation of the National Patient Safety Foundation (NPSF) by the American Medical Association (AMA). The Veterans Health Administration (VHA) undertook sweeping changes in its health-care system to reduce medical errors. It established centres of excellence to foster the much-needed, multidisciplinary research and design of safer systems of medical care.

A significant proportion of leading scientific research work on patient safety and medical error reduction in complex systems has also come from European researchers.

In the UK, there is now a system in place to record and monitor medical errors, near misses, and adverse events occurring both in the National Health Service (NHS) and within private health-care providers' institutions. In the past, the NHS concentrated on dealing with individual errors rather than the environment that predisposed people to err.

In everyday life, we all employ a common human defence mechanism whenever we think of the unthinkable, which is that 'it will never happen to me'. Medical errors and adverse events do happen, sometimes when we least expect them. If errors could be predicted, they would be avoided altogether. Medical errors do produce major psychological trauma in doctors as much as in those members of staff who witness them. This psychological damage may last for a very long time, sometimes for life. Members of the medical profession and their patients should maintain a good doctor-patient relationship, honesty, and good communication. Following the occurrence of medical errors, different organisations, with different hierarchies and responsibilities, will be drawn together to deal with the *aftermath*. These organisations have different expertise, different priorities, and different jurisdiction.

It is essential to have in place organised help and support for the doctors and those team members involved in the occurrence of medical errors. This support should be available locally in the initial stages of the aftermath. Medical defence organisations look after their members' interests whatever the circumstances, and therefore, membership to these organisations is highly recommended. The General Medical Council (GMC) in the UK does police the conduct and other activities of doctors and, together with other agencies of state, may offer help and advice to individual doctors in an effort to rehabilitate and retrain such doctors. The General Medical Council actively encourages activities which improve self-regulation, continuing medical education, continuing professional development, and does supervise the revalidation and licensing of doctors.

Reading this book will be a step forward in the understanding of various factors which contribute to the occurrence of medical errors and adverse events and ways in which to deal with the aftermath. Prevention is better than cure.

Acknowledgements

This book would not have been produced without the encouragement and support of some of my *consultant colleagues* in the Directorate of Anaesthesia and Critical Care at the William Harvey Hospital, Ashford, Kent, East Kent Hospitals University NHS Foundation Trust, UK. I also wish to extend my gratitude to *Ms Sharon Blackmore*, secretary to the Directorate of Anaesthesia and Critical Care, for introducing me to many medical representatives working in the Kent area, who expressed interest in the book.

May I extend my appreciation to: *Mr Andrew Grice*, editor of Minerva Press (UK); *Ms Grace Chisholm*, executive editor of Pentland Books; *Ms Carol Biss*, managing director at The Book Guild Limited; *Prof. Rory Shaw*, ex-chairman of National Patients Agency; and last but not least, *Mr Arnold J. Simanowitz* of Action for Victims of Medical Accidents organisation, UK, who gave me *encouraging testimonials* about the book. It has been a long while since my last contact with these *notables,* but their appraisal of the manuscript gave me hope of getting this book on the shelves. Finally, I am grateful to *Linda* and *Barbara*, my daughters, for helping me with computer-based activities related to this publication.

Chapter 1

Definitions of Terms Used in the Text

Adverse Event or Incident: 'an unintended injury that is caused, at least in part, by medical management (rather than by underlying disease) that prolongs the hospitalisation of a patient or produces a measurable disability at the time of discharge, or both of these'.

It should be noted that not every medical error produces injury to a patient and not every adverse event is a result of a medical error.

The Bolam Test—the required standard of medical care: In the UK, the legally required standard of medical care a doctor generally owes to a patient is based on the Bolam Test. The Bolam Test arose from a case where it was argued that the hospital was vicariously liable for the carelessness of a doctor who gave electroconvulsive therapy (*ECT*) to Mr Bolam without administering a muscle relaxant or restraining the convulsive movements to prevent injury. Mr Bolam sustained a fractured jaw during the procedure, and the case became known as the Bolam vs Friern Barnet Health Management Committee in 1957. The court sought the opinion of other doctors who worked in this area of medical practice, and they supported the actions of the accused doctor. Mr Bolam lost the case.

The key point that arose from this case was not the clinical situation and the adverse event which followed it, but it was the idea that the standard of care should be measured by other professionals who normally undertake the role of the defendant.

In the words of the judge, and I quote, 'A doctor is not guilty of negligence if he/she has acted in accordance with a practice accepted as proper by a responsible body of medical men and women skilled in that particular art.' Under English law, the Bolam Test was slightly modified following the case of Bolitho in 1997, which now means that an English court is not bound to hold that a particular practice is acceptable simply because there is a "responsible body of medical opinion which supports it" unless that body of opinion can demonstrate such opinion has a logical basis and that the experts have directed their minds to the question of comparative risks and benefits to reach a defensible conclusion.'

Clinical Governance: defined as 'a framework through which the National Health Service (NHS) organisations in the UK are accountable for continuously improving the quality of their services and safeguarding high standards of health care by creating an environment in which excellence in clinical care will flourish'.

Critical Incident: defined as 'any episode of patient care in which specific actions by a doctor or any other medical practitioner has specific beneficial or detrimental effects on a patient'. The term *critical* simply means that, very likely, the medical practitioner's actions were directly responsible for the effects observed in the patient. Cooper et al defined a critical incident in anesthesiology as, 'an occurrence that could have led, if not corrected in time, or did lead to an undesirable outcome ranging from increased length of stay in hospital or to death of the patient'.

Deposition: defined as 'an out of court testimony of a witness recorded in writing under oath or affirmation'.

Disability: 'a physical or mental state resulting from an injury or injuries, or abnormal development which limits normal activities by the patient. Disability can be temporary or permanent'.

Discovery: 'a process whereby the parties and their legal teams attempt to uncover, review, and evaluate all evidence having any bearing on the facts of the case'.

Duty of Care: 'reasonable care which avoids acts or omissions which one can reasonably foresee would be likely to injure a person directly affected by these acts or omissions'.

Expert Witness: 'a medical or other professional whose evidence to a court may prove that the defendant violated the applicable standard of care in treating the patient'.

Correspondingly, an expert may testify as to the compliance of the defendant with standards of care, the appropriateness of decisions and actions, and in some cases, perhaps the inevitability of the patient's outcome even with the best of care.

Fallibility: 'quality of being fallible, i.e. liability to err'.

Informed Consent: 'voluntary and continuing permission of a patient or legal authority to receive specified medical treatment based on an adequate knowledge of purpose, nature, likely effects, and risks of that treatment, including the likelihood of its success or failure, and any alternatives to it'.

Medical Error: 'an unintended act of commission or omission or one that does not achieve its intended outcome; or an unanticipated negative consequence of a medical intervention or non-intervention here called commission or omission'. Unanticipated negative consequence of a medical intervention is defined as 'patient reactions which increase morbidity or pain or results in death of a patient'. Medical interventions include diagnosis, test procedures, and prescribing drugs, among others.

Medical Device: 'any health-care product, excluding drugs, which is used for a patient in the diagnosis, treatment, prevention, or alleviation of illness or injury'.

Medical Equipment: 'the necessary article or machinery for a medical purpose'.

Medical Mistake: 'an unanticipated *negative* consequence of medical intervention'.

Medical Negligence: 'care that falls below the standard expected of a doctor in his/her community or a failure to meet the standard of practice of an average qualified doctor practicing in the same specialty under the same conditions on a similar patient'.

Negligence occurs not merely when there is an error, but when the degree of error exceeds the expected norm. The presence of error is necessary but not sufficient condition for the determination of negligence. Medical negligence is a composite of three essential elements: *First is duty of care.* The plaintiff (accuser) must show that the defendant owed him/her a duty of care. *Second is breach of duty.* The plaintiff must show that the defendant (accused), here the doctor, breached this duty of care by failing to provide the required standard of care. *Third is actual cause of harm.* The plaintiff must prove that this failure to provide the required standard of care by the doctor actually caused him/her the harm.

Post-traumatic Stress Disorder: 'a process which follows the occurrence of a disastrous experience by an individual or group of individuals; manifested by the occurrence of nightmares, major sleep disturbance, phobias of places, including workplace, or anything associated with the disaster'. These difficulties are referred to as post-traumatic stress disorder.

Professionalism: 'is the acceptable practice of an occupation which one professes to be skilled in and to follow'. Professionalism can be practiced as a vocation in which a professed knowledge of some department of learning or science is used in its application to the affairs of others or in the practice of an art founded upon it.

Re-validation (or Re-certification): 'is an ending examination of the roles, rights, and responsibilities of the medical profession'. It is a process whereby doctors demonstrate to their peers, patients, as well as to their employers that they are worthy and fit to be on the medical register of the General Medical Council in the UK.

Self-Regulation: 'a process whereby the clinical work of individual doctors can be judged by clinicians with at least the same level of specialist knowledge and experience as the doctor concerned'. Under this scheme, senior doctors appraise colleagues in other hospitals who work in the same specialty. Under this principle, the Parliament of the UK gives doctors the privilege of professional independence embodied in self-regulation.

Stress: 'is a body's reaction to actual or anticipated difficulties in life, difficulties which may be related to daily activities or more complex and unusual situations'. People do need a certain amount of stress to perform at their best, but too much stress produces many negative effects.

System: 'is a set of elements interacting to achieve a shaped aim, or a methodically arranged set of ideas, methods, or procedures to achieve a specified outcome'.

References

1. Lisby et al., How Are Medication Errors Defined? A Systematic Literature Review of Definitions and Characteristics, *International Journal for Quality In Health Care*, 2010, **22**(6), 507-18.
2. Naomi Engel, Jennifer Dmetrichuk, and Anne-Marie Shanks, Medical Professionalism: Can It and Should It Be Measured? *British Medical Journal*, 2009, 161-2.
3. Green M., Zick A., Makaul G., Defining Professionalism from the Perspective of Patients, Physicians, and Nurses, *Acad. Med.*, 2009, **84**, 556-73.
4. Levenson R., Dewar S., Shepherd S., Understanding Doctors: Harnessing Professionalism, King's Fund and Royal College of Physicians, 2008.
5. Report of a Working Party of the Royal College of Physicians of London 2005, Royal College of Physicians, Doctors in Society: Medical Professionalism in a Changing World, Royal College of Physicians, 2005.
6. Nicola Woolcock and M. Henderson, Blundering Hospitals 'Kill 40,000 Every Year', *The Times* (UK), 13 August, 2004, No. 68153, *www.timesonline.co.uk*
7. Graham Buckley, Revalidation Is the Answer, *British Medical Journal*, 1999, **319**, 1145-6.
8. Timothy P. Hofer, What Is an Error? *http://www.acponline.org/journals/ecp/novedec00/hofer.htm*
9. Donald M. Berwick, Lucian L. Leape, Reducing Errors in Medicine, *British Medical Journal*, 1999, **319**, 136-7.
10. Zosia Kmietowicz, All UK Doctors to Be Required to Prove Competence, *British Medical Journal*, 1999, **318**, 482.
11. Nic Paton, Adverse Incidents, *Hospital Doctor* (UK), July 1999, 4.

12. Lucian L. Leape, Incidence of Adverse Events and Negligence in Hospitalised Patients, *The New England Journal of Medicine*, 1991, **324**(6), 377-84.
13. R. J. Asher, Critical questions; Critical Incidents; Critical answers, *The Lancet*, 1988, 1373-4.
14. Terry Mizrahi, Managing Medical Mistakes; Ideology, Insularity, and Accountability Among Interns in Training, *Soc. Sci. Med.*, 1984, **19**(2), 135-46.
15. Cooper et al., Critical Incidents in Medical Care, *Anesthesiology*, 1978, **49**, 406.

Chapter 2

Training of Doctors and Practising Medicine as a Profession

Teaching medical undergraduates about medical errors was, until recently, patchy and very limited here in the UK. Experience of such occurrence has also been limited and partial, because students are always shadowed by their tutors. Therefore, the impact of errors is not as dramatic as it is later on in their careers.

Graduation from medical training abruptly forces new and young, inexperienced doctors into a world in which they become responsible for life-and-death decisions. Sometimes, these decisions have catastrophic consequences for their patients. At other times, their decisions are detrimental to patients, prolonging pain and creating problems where there were none before and aggravating the healing process. The training of doctors may not address worries about harm done to their patients, and they are not prepared for the death of their patients. So the inexperienced, most vulnerable doctors find themselves in a very difficult situation when faced with the occurrence of a medical error.

It is the current trend to worry about possible legal action by the patients or their relatives even if defending such action is the responsibility of tutors and other authorities.

Medical Oaths and Codes

The main intention of a medical oath seems to be to declare the core values of professional integrity, including traditional moral virtues such as compassion and honesty. Oaths also provide moral orientation through rule-like precepts and prohibitions from which generalities the practitioner is left to infer or extrapolate to the specifics of everyday practice. Medical codes, on the other hand, seek to clarify the means by which such moral ends can be achieved by offering guidance for everyday practice, outlining applicability in exemplary cases, together with grounds for identifying exceptions. Affirmation of an ethical code by means of an oath, therefore, permits the oath to contain, within its remit, a supplementary field of guidance.

The Hippocratic Oath

The Hippocratic Oath comes from the writings of Hippocrates, a Greek physician who influenced the last *2500 years* of medical practice. Hippocrates was a father of medicine and his writings are better known as *Hippocratic Corpus*. They are multi-author volumes with internal inconsistencies, abrupt changes of style and tone, and incompatible world views.

Here in the UK, the General Medical Council (GMC) issued its professional code, and together with the British Medical Association (BMA), the Royal colleges, and other organisations, published a document on the 'core values' of medical practice. The BMA drafted a new Hippocratic Oath on behalf of the World Medical Association, which is reproduced below.

"The practice of medicine is a privilege which carries important responsibilities. All doctors should observe the core values of the profession which centre on the duty to help sick people and to avoid harm. I promise that my medical knowledge will be used to benefit people's health. They are my first concern. I will listen to them and provide the best care I can. I will be honest, respectful, and compassionate towards patients. In emergencies, I will do my best to help anyone in medical need. I will make every effort to ensure that the rights of all patients are respected, including those of vulnerable groups who lack means of making their needs known, be it through immaturity, medical incapacity, imprisonment or detention or other circumstance. My professional judgement will be exercised as independently as possible and not be influenced by political pressure, nor by factors such as the social standing of the patient. I will not put personal profit or advancement above my duty to patients. I will recognise the special value of human life, but also know the prolongation of human life is not the only aim of health care. Where abortion is permitted, I agree that it should take place only within the ethical and legal framework. I will not provide treatments which are pointless or harmful, or which an informed and competent patient refuses. I will ensure patients receive the information and support they want to make decisions about disease prevention and improvement of their health. I will answer as truthfully as I can and respect patients' decisions unless that puts others at risk of harm. If I cannot agree with their requests, I will explain why.

If my patients have limited mental awareness, I will still encourage them to participate in decisions as much as they feel able and willing to do so. I will do my best to maintain confidentiality about all patients. If there are overriding reasons which prevent my keeping a patient's confidentiality, I will explain them. I will recognise the limits of my knowledge and seek advice from colleagues when necessary. I will acknowledge my mistakes. I will do my best to keep myself and colleagues informed of new developments and ensure that poor standards or bad practices are exposed to those who can improve them. I will show respect for all those with whom I work and be ready to share my knowledge by teaching others what I know. I will use my training and professional standing to improve the community in which I work. I will treat patients equitably and support a fair and humane distribution of health resources. I will try to influence positively authorities whose policies harm public health. I will oppose policies which breach internationally accepted standards of human rights. I will strive to change laws which are contrary to patients' interests or to my professional ethics."

The American Medical Association, in 1997, commemorated the 150th anniversary of its 1847 Code of Ethics with an exhaustive debate on the relevance of oaths and codes to modern medical practice. Re-fashioning health care in order to contain costs in many countries has precipitated rapid flux in the social relationships of medical practice. Doctors are no longer in a simple clinical relationship with their patients. The structure of health services now involves them in many other tasks, some of which may entail conflicting responsibilities. Funding organisations and managers increasingly influence the nature and extent of care which can be provided. At the same time, health care has become multidisciplinary in nature and multi-agency in delivery. Scientific advances and new technological capabilities throw up difficult and sometimes bizarre moral predicaments.

All these changes make for greater moral complexity in everyday practice. The medical profession has to face hard choices in patient care and re-examine its own role in health care. It has to look again at the nature of its own values.

The Hippocratic Oath has been re-examined afresh for moral guidance. The oath entails making a covenant with other members of the profession to share knowledge freely, to respect one's teachers, and to behave towards patients according to the *Hippocratic Code*, the text of which follows:

"I will follow that system of regimen which, according to my ability and judgement, I consider for the benefit of my patients, and abstain from whatever is deleterious and mischievous. I will give no deadly medicine to any one if asked, nor suggest any such counsel; and in like manner I will not give to a woman a pessary to produce abortion. With purity and with holiness, I will pass my life and practice my art. I will not cut persons labouring under the stone, but will leave this to be done by men who are practitioners of this work. Into whatever house I enter, I will go into them for the benefit of the sick and I will abstain from every voluntary act of mischief and corruption, and further, from the seduction of females or males, of freshmen and slaves. Whatever, in connection with it, I see or hear, in the life of men, which ought not to be spoken of abroad, I will not divulge, as reckoning that all such should be kept secret."

The Changing Oath

Problems and controversies surround the textual authenticity and meaning of the original *Hippocratic Oath*. It is probably that only a minority of doctors swore the oath in ancient Greece. Some of its prohibitions fly in the face of what was happening in clinical practice in ancient Greece, like surgery, abortion, and tolerance of infanticide. Those administering the oath during succeeding centuries have taken it on themselves to omit, add to, and change its clauses. There are many incongruities in the original oath that make it difficult to apply to present day medical care.

Many modern institutions bypass the problem altogether by administering oaths which are entirely modern in content, but are titled Hippocratic. Over 50 per cent of medical schools in the UK and almost all those in the USA administer an oath of some kind, mostly at graduation but occasionally earlier, and a few at the onset of medical studies. Some use a modernised version of the Hippocratic Oath or of the *Prayer of Maimonides*. Others use the *Declaration of Geneva* (printed below), and others still use their own institutional oath. Oath-taking processes also differ, with some schools asking for graduates' affirmation by signature, and others reading the oath out or reciting it during the graduation ceremony.

Declaration of Geneva

"At the time of being admitted as a member of my profession, I solemnly pledge myself to consecrate my life to the service of humanity; I will give to my teachers the respect and gratitude which is their due; I will practice my profession with conscience and dignity. The health of those in my care will be my first consideration; I will respect the secrets that are confided in me even after the patient has died; I will maintain by all the means in my power, the honour and the noble traditions of my profession. My colleagues will be my sisters and brothers; I will not permit considerations of age, disease or disability, creed, ethnic origin, gender, nationality, political affiliation, race, sexual orientation or social standing, to intervene between my duty and my patient. I will maintain the utmost respect for human life from its beginning, even under threat, and I will not use my specialist knowledge contrary to the laws of humanity. I make these promises solemnly, freely, and upon my honour."

Pan-professional Oath

The American Academy of Arts and Science instigated a trans-Atlantic initiative to create a shared ethical code for all health carers. This pan-professional oath could engender a positive degree of moral cohesion between all caring professions, across institutional boundaries, influencing perhaps even the organisation of health care. It is hoped a single oath for all health-care professions could heal split loyalties and ameliorate existing moral tensions in health care.

The intention is honourable but no one should underestimate the difficulty of the task. Such an oath provides an inclusive opportunity for health-care workers from different walks of life to speak with one voice for the benefit of patients.

Career training in the National Health Service (NHS) in the UK

The overwhelming majority of the training network is made up of doctors most of whom fulfil a clinical commitment as well as perform their educational role. The trainers' hierarchy is from the supervising consultant to the postgraduate dean. These officials ensure a continuous supply of well-informed and experienced doctors who support trainees and junior doctors. They establish and maintain the essential links between the three basic elements of medical education, namely, the universities, Royal colleges, and the National Health Service (NHS). Some deaneries moved away from reliance on clinical staff to run training and appointed full-time educationists who advised on curriculum development, methods of assessment, and monitoring the quality of medical education.

Postgraduate dean—He/she is the most powerful individual in the trainees' education. There were twenty-three deans, each one looking after what is called a deanery, but there have been some changes in this cadre. There is also a Postgraduate Dean of the Armed Forces. It is a full-time job for most and requires them to stand aside from their clinical commitments.

The dean heads a team that oversees the entire range of doctors' postgraduate training. His/her deputy or associate postgraduate dean oversees the regional advisor for postgraduate education (in some areas) and the clinical tutor.

The postgraduate dean is appointed by the universities and National Health Service (NHS) executive in England and Wales, and by the Scottish Council for Postgraduate Medical and Dental Education in Scotland. In Northern Ireland, these appointments are made by the Department of Health. They are fund-holders for postgraduate training. Their primary task is to make sure the training system produces enough trainees at each grade and in every specialty to meet agreed workforce needs and for tomorrow's consultants to have solid professional and specialist training. They also promote lifelong learning for incumbent consultants, thus ensuring that everyone involved in the trainees' education remains competent and up to date.

Specific duties include liaison with the Royal colleges on training requirements and standards, inspecting training programmes and individual training posts, identifying and supporting those trainees who need help, developing opportunities for flexible training, and developing systems for appraisal and assessment. Deans do not remain remote from the trainees.

They go out to meet them and their trainers to discuss issues relating to training and workload.

Deputy Associate Dean—This education official liaises with the universities in appointing deputies and associates. The post is sessional, usually filled by a consultant who has day-to-day clinical care role. He/she supports the dean for specific roles such as supervising the transition from medical student to pre-registration foundation doctor and development of flexible training. Some deaneries appoint regional advisors on postgraduate medical and dental education who address areas such as curriculum educational methods.

Clinical Tutors—Clinical tutors are appointed by the postgraduate deans, and many are given the post of director of postgraduate medical education by their employers, the NHS trusts. This is a dual job description and a two-way accountability which helps to underpin what is largely a bridge-building role. Clinical tutors provide links between the often conflicting interests of education and service, of trust and academia, and sometimes, trainee and trainer. They facilitate communication between the deanery, the university, the employer (trust) and individual trainees and trainers. They monitor educational standards in all the deaneries, check that assessment and appraisal systems are in place, and make sure training programmes do not suffer neglect. Clinical tutors are also responsible for the day-to-day working of the postgraduate educational centres and the courses they offer, including those covering generic skills such as communication and other predictable clinical topics.

Regional Advisors—They are appointed by the Royal colleges to represent the interests of specialties at the regional level. Their strategic role involves making sure optimal standard of training in their specialty is maintained. They sit on and often chair specialty training committees and those which appoint new trainees. Regional advisors have strong influence on the content of trainee programmes and on the validation of consultant posts, thus ensuring the appointment of high calibre trainers. They get involved in the assessment of trainees including the formal annual review. They are available to advise and counsel individual trainees. They oversee the training programme directors, college tutors, associate college tutors (in some specialties) and supervisors.

Training Programme Directors—Their role involves organising and overseeing training placements in specialties, liaison with personnel departments, coordinating new training posts, and getting involved in assessments. They help trainees get work experience placements and offer advice and guidance to newly qualified doctors with work-related and personal problems and worries.

College Tutors—These are consultants who provide the link between the Royal colleges and individual employers (NHS trusts). They help to implement the strategic work of regional advisors. They provide support and career advice for trainees and make sure the postgraduate training in their specialty follows the requirements and standards of the college concerned. Their specific duties include inspection of trainees' posts in their particular specialty, making sure all supervising consultants are adequately trained for the job. They organise teaching for examinations, supervise logbook keeping and carry out appraisals. They prepare for the regular formal assessment visits to the trusts by the relevant Royal college officials and prepare reports afterwards.

Associate College Tutors—These are junior doctors in training who help college tutors to organise teaching rotas and prepare for Royal college visits. They canvass and give feedback to college tutors on their trainee opinions.

Supervising Consultants—These consultants have the greatest day-to-day interaction with individual trainees. They oversee the content of training programmes, making sure every individual trainee has the experience needed to progress to the next stage of their career. Often, this means identifying and overcoming barriers in the way of practical experiences. Supervising consultants monitor the progress of training by assessing that which has been achieved thus far and setting the next goals to be tackled. Such goals could be audit projects or experience of procedures. These goals are chosen according to the trainee's aims and specialty. In many cases, the consultant supervisor acts as a mentor, providing help and guidance to the trainee on career and personal issues.

Committees and Panels—There are the Specialty Training Committee, Appointments Panels, and the Annual Review Panel. Trainee doctors experience scrutiny by teams of consultants as they go through appointment panels. They must go through the Annual Review Panel (ARP) before they progress to the next stage of higher specialist training. The Specialty Training Committee (STC) decides on the trainee's rotations and other training issues. A trainee may observe that the same names and faces tend to feature on many of these bodies. It is not unusual for the local Annual Review Panel (ARP) and the Specialty Training Committee (STC) in a given specialty to be chaired by the same consultant, often the regional advisor.

Job titles can be confusing. Clinical tutors and College tutors have totally different duties, responsibilities, and lines of accountability. Many Clinical tutors also hold the job title of postgraduate medical education director given by employing trusts.

Professionalism and the Medical Profession

A profession is defined as 'the occupation which one professes to be skilled in and to follow—a vocation in which a professed knowledge of some department of learning or science is used in its application to the affairs of others, or in practice of an art founded upon it'. In a wider sense, profession can be defined as 'any calling or occupation by which a person habitually earns his/her living'. This definition, however, does not adequately describe the complexity of modern professions.

Lack of literature on professionalism available to doctors and the absence of relevant material in the curriculum of most medical schools has hampered the proper understanding of professionalism. Most doctors do not understand the obligations they must fulfil to satisfy public expectations and maintain professional status. Doctors would meet their obligations if they understand their origins and their nature. Therefore professionalism must be taught.

Doctors fill two overlapping roles of the healer and the professional. Many doctors feel that fulfilling the role of a healer is sufficient and do not willingly accept professional obligations. For example, the healer is under no obligation to sit on audit committees or to engage in other administrative activities, but the professional must. Society requires that there must be an organisational framework within which the services of the healer are dispensed. In the modern world, professional status is granted by the state and defined by laws outlining licensing and in the charters and regulations of the various certifying bodies. It can be modified or withdrawn if society is not satisfied with the performance of its professionals.

In the UK, the General Medical Council's approach to professionalism and self-regulation is a response to the rapidly changing relation of all professions to society and is designed to allow medicine to meet new societal demands and expectations. Professionalism in the modern world should address the following important points:

1) The importance of independence (autonomy) which depends on these three pillars: *expertise*, *ethics*, and *service*.

2) The importance of trust between patient and doctor and between the profession and society.

3) The availability of leaders to provide the much-needed role models.

In the UK and the USA, governments granted the medical profession the right to self-regulation. Autonomy is given on the understanding that professionals will put the welfare of both the patient and society above their own and that they will be governed by a code of ethics. Professionalism is an ideal which, if pursued, should enable striving doctors to reach even higher levels of performance. Medical schools, teaching hospitals, and those professionals responsible for continuing medical education (CME) should teach professionalism as a subject formally identified in the curriculum. The material to be taught will change in different cultures and certainly with time. The teaching of professionalism should include several components.

The main *components* of teaching professionalism are as follows:

1. A clear definition of professionalism and its characteristics.
2. Inclusion of identifiable educational content in the undergraduate medical school curriculum devoted to professionalism, reinforced in postgraduate programmes and in continuing medical education. This subject should be part of the evaluation of all medical students.
3. The concept that to be a professional is not a *right* but a *privilege* with a long history and tradition of healing as a service.
4. The separate but linked concepts of the doctor as a healer and the doctor as a professional and the fact that society uses professional status as a means of organising the delivery of services.
5. Promotion of professionalism as an ideal to be pursued, emphasising its inherent moral value. The concept of *altruism* (unselfishness) and *calling* must be highlighted as essential to professionalism.

6. An understanding that proper behaviour is essential for the healer to function fully and to maintain the trust of patients and society.
7. Improve on knowledge of codes of ethics governing the conduct of both the healer and the professional as well as the philosophical and historical derivations of these codes.
8. The essential nature of the autonomy of the individual doctor along with the legitimate limitations that have always existed. The degree of autonomy will vary in different societies, but a minimum is required for a doctor to exercise the necessary independent judgement to best serve the patient.
9. The nature of the collective autonomy of the profession along with its legitimate and inherent limitations.
10. Relevant material drawn from sociology, philosophy, economics, political science, and medical ethics as related to professionalism, including interpretations of both the historical course of events and doctors' behaviour that are critical of the medical profession. The profession must not be allowed to build and maintain its own myths while avoiding ideas challenging them.
11. The link between professional status and obligations to society that must be fulfilled to maintain public trust. These obligations must be explicitly outlined and included in the teaching. They include obligations to know and be guided by the applicable codes of ethics and national as well as regional laws, to participate in more effective and transparent self-regulation; to address health issues of concern to society; to maintain competence throughout one's medical career and to be prepared to be fully accountable for all decisions taken; to expand and ensure the integrity of the medical knowledge base by supporting science in the broadest sense; to insist on the maintenance of sufficient individual and professional autonomy to enable the doctor to act in the best interests of the patient; and finally, to be governed by professional standards of conduct no matter what role is being filled.

In summary, the following points on *professionalism* should be noted:

- That professional status is not an inherent right but is granted by society.
- That maintenance of professional status depends on the public's belief that professionals are trustworthy.

- That to remain trustworthy, professionals must meet the obligations expected by society.
- That the substance of professionalism should be taught at all levels of medical education as part of the profession's response to changing societal expectations.

References

1. Varkey et al., A Patient Safety Curriculum for Graduate Education: Results from a Needs Assessment of Education and Patient Safety Experts, *American Journal of Medical Quality*, 2009, **24**, 214-21.
2. Singh et al., Building Learning Practices with Self-empowered Teams for Improving Patient Safety, *Journal of Health Management*, 2006, **8**, 91-118.
3. I. Loefler, Hippocratic Ideals Are Dead, *British Medical Journal*, **324**, 463.
4. John Fabre, Hip, Hip, Hippocrates—Extracts from 'The Hippocratic Doctor', *British Medical Journal*, 1997, **315**, 1669-70.
5. Brian Hurwitz and Ruth Richardson, Swearing to Care: The Resurgence in Medical Oaths, *British Medical Journal*, 1997, **315**, 1671-3.
6. General Medical Council, Training Doctors in the Future, *General Medical Council News*, 1997, Issue 2.
7. Sylvia R. Cruess and Richard L. Cruess, Professionalism Must Be Taught, *British Medical Journal*, 1997, **315**, 1674-6.

Chapter 3

Classification of Medical Errors

Types of errors will vary according to the medical specialty, the task at hand, and the people involved, both patients and medical staff. J. Cooper et al. classified anaesthetic errors as technical, judgemental, monitoring, and vigilance. These errors, with the exception of technical ones, are based on psychological processes of judgement, attention, and memory. Cruves and Fries discussed *diagnostic errors*, which they classified as those due to lack of adequate history, errors of omission, misleading test results, and errors due to problems with physical examination. Errors may also be classified according to the most effective way of preventing them, e.g., by providing standing orders and by clinical algorithms.

Lucian L. Leape et al. in their Harvard Medical Practice Study 11 on the 'nature of adverse events in hospitalised patients', in the state of New York, USA, (New England Journal of Medicine, 1991) grouped medical errors as follows:

Performance errors, in which inadequate preparation of patients before procedure, technical errors, inadequate monitoring of patients after procedure, use of inappropriate or outmoded form of therapy, avoidable delay in treatment, and the doctor or other professional practicing outside area of expertise were some of the factors involved.

Diagnostic errors, in which failure to use indicated tests, failure to act on results or findings, use of outmoded or inappropriate diagnostic tests, avoidable delay in diagnosis, and physician or other professional practicing outside area of expertise are important factors.

Drug treatment errors, where error in dosage or method of use, failure to recognise possible antagonistic or complementary drug interactions, inadequate follow-up of therapy, use of inappropriate drugs, avoidable delay in treatment, and physician or other personnel practicing outside area of expertise are factors.

System-based errors, in which defective equipment or supplies, inadequate or total lack of equipment or supplies, inadequate monitoring system, inadequate reporting or communications, inadequate training or supervision of physician or other personnel, delay in provision or scheduling of service, inadequate staffing, and inadequate functioning of hospital services are contributory factors.

Prevention-based errors, which include failure to take precautions to prevent accidental injury, failure to use indicated tests, failure to act on results of tests or findings, use of inappropriate or outmoded diagnostic tests, avoidable delay in treatment, and physician or other personnel practicing outside their area of expertise.

References

1. M. Bromiley, Have You Ever Made a Mistake? *Bulletin of RCoA,* March 2008, Issue 48.
2. Bell D., Recurrent Wrong-route Drug Error—a Professional Shame, *Anaesthesia,* 2007, **62**, 541-4.
3. Merry A. et al., Prospective Assessment of a New Anaesthetic Drug Administration System Designed to Improve Safety, *Anesthesiology,* 2006, **106**, A138
4. Charles Vincent, Reducing Error in Medicine, *British Medical Journal Conference,* March 2000.
5. Professor Carlo Fonseka, To Err Was Fatal, *British Medical Journal,* 1996, **313**, 1640-2.
6. Lucian L. Leape, The Nature of Adverse Events and Negligence in Hospitalised Patients, *The New England Journal of Medicine,* 1991, **324**(6), 377-84.
7. Merry A. F. et al., Anaesthetists, Errors in Drug Administration and the Law, *New Zealand Medical Journal,* 1995, **108**, 185-7.

8. C. A. Vincent, Research into Medical Accidents—A Case of Negligence? *British Medical Journal*, 1989, **299**, 1150-3.
9. Prof. Chris Bulstrode, On Course to Change the Face of Training, *Hospital Doctor* (UK), February 1999, 38-40.

Chapter 4

Incidence of Medical Errors and Adverse Events in the UK and USA

Health-care systems have checks and safeguards to reduce the occurrence of medical errors and adverse events. They aim at avoiding and preventing adverse events or injury through the health care they provide. However, despite these interventions, almost 10 per cent of hospital patients experience an adverse event during their care and yet about 40 per cent of these events are preventable, (see Leape L., Berwick. D, Journal of American Medical Association, 2005, **293**, 238490).

Although the use of a variety of indicators has resulted in more attention to procedural checks such as prevention of wrong site, wrong patient, wrong procedure events, there is little evidence for a significant reduction in the number of adverse events (says Laurent Degos and colleagues, Breaking the Mould in Patient Safety, *British Medical Journal,* 2009, **339**, 82-4).

Iatrogenic adverse reactions may develop from a wide array of modern diagnostic or therapeutic practices. Modern medicine has enormous power to cure or palliate, but serious side effects still occur. Adverse events can follow risky procedures or occur as honest and legitimate errors of judgement in which the doctor acted in good faith, made a decision that turned out not to be the best, but involved no negligence or substandard care. Adverse events can result from decisions and actions by the doctor where he/she is, to some degree, obviously culpable of malpractice or negligence.

In Britain, in 2000, it was estimated that 850,000 adverse events occurred in the hospital sector of the NHS each year, and according to the National

Patients Agency, adverse events contribute to an estimated 72,000 deaths every year. In one study, the most common medical mistakes were errors in administering anaesthetics and in prescribing and giving drugs. Since 1985, there were fourteen blunders involving the cancer drug Vincristine, eleven of which were fatal. Details can be found in Department of Health document, *An Organisation with a Memory* published in 2000. Up to date statistics for the UK are available at the Department of Health or National Patient Safety Agency.

In the USA, medical errors have been estimated to cause between 44,000 and 98,000 deaths in hospital-based services a year. More than a million injuries are caused by errors each year, according to Wikipedia sources. Apparently a conservative estimate by both the Institute of Medicine and Health Grades reports was four hundred thousand to a million and two hundred thousand error-induced deaths between the 1996 and 2006 period.

A study carried out in my trust, East Kent Hospitals University NHS Foundation Trust, UK, between October 2003 and December 2004 came up with the following findings. Most reported *adverse clinical incidents* were in the order as follows:

Drug errors;
Errors in communication;
General accident management;
Missing patients' medical notes;
Errors relating to blood transfusion;
Incorrect data in patients' notes;
Equipment malfunction;
Missing or lack of equipments;
Inappropriate treatment;
Inadequate consent;
Incorrect or incomplete operating theatre lists;
Wrong patient (i.e., patients incorrectly identified);
Delayed diagnostic reports;
Poor nursing care leading to patients developing pressure sores and infections.

In this study, the number of adverse clinical incidents by directorate for the same period was as follows:

General medicine (including psychiatry) had by far the highest number of clinical incidents, two to three times more than most of the other directorates. This was followed by Women's Health (Obstetrics and Gynaecology); General Surgery (GS); Anaesthesia (including Critical Care Medicine); Trauma and Orthopaedics (T & Orth.); Pathology; Accident and Emergency (A&E); Child Health (Paediatrics); Head and Neck (ENT); Out-patient Department (OPD); and Pharmacy.

A high incidence of errors in the medical profession may be due to the following reasons:

1. *Culture of 'Blame' in medical practice*, the concept of infallibility, is built or developed by the powerful emphasis on perfection both in diagnosis and treatment and the doctor's perception of error as a failure of character. Doctors are expected to function without making errors. There is strong pressure to intellectual dishonesty created by the need to be infallible.

2. *Cultivation of a norm of high standard*—'if you are responsible for everything that happens to a patient, it follows that you are responsible for every error that occurs.' Note how absurd this conclusion is as it assumes that doctors have power to control all aspects of patient care!

The organisation of medical practice, particularly hospital-based medical practice, penetrates these norms. Errors are reluctantly admitted or discussed among doctors. Most doctors typically feel that admission of error will lead to censure or increased surveillance or, worse, that their colleagues will regard them as incompetent or careless. Doctors are devastated by errors that harm or kill their patients.

In its annual state health care report of 2008, the Healthcare Commission (now the Care Quality Commission) stated that *many incidents* where patients were harmed or where there were near misses in England *were not being reported*. Errors that had led to patients being harmed included incorrect diagnosis, wrong doses of medications, surgeons operating on the wrong part of the body or performing wrong operations, and missing patient notes. Lessons were not being learnt and problems persisted. There was lack of progress in the previous five years.

One in ten (10 per cent) patients admitted into hospitals were to suffer an error and 50 per cent of these errors could have been avoided. Only half of the NHS trusts were complying with patient safety standards, and there had been little improvement. The report said that too few incidents were reported to the National Patient Safety Agency (NPSA), with particular problem in primary care, where doctors and nurses reported almost no errors, although the majority of patients' care is delivered by general practitioners (GPs). In 2008, it is estimated, there were about *600 errors every day in primary care*, a figure disputed by the Department of Health (DoH) and the British Medical Association (BMA).

The National Patient Safety Agency (NPSA) received *959,000* reports of incidents of medical errors in 2007/8, and worryingly, this report says 7 per cent of hospital trusts and 13 per cent of primary care trusts did not report any incidents.

The extent of the problem and incidence of medical errors in the USA was estimated at one million potentially preventable medical errors, of which one hundred and twenty thousand died each year in the early 1990s. At that time, there was reliance on self-reporting by doctors. Prof. Lucian Leape stated that reliance on self-reporting missed almost 90 per cent of doctors' errors.

A study done in 1984 in New York State showed errors to occur in 3.7 per cent of hospitalised patients, and 1 per cent of these errors were due to *negligence*, 70.5 per cent of errors gave rise to *temporary disability* lasting less than six months, 2.6 per cent of errors caused *permanent disability,* and 3.6 per cent of errors led to *deaths* of patients. One was to assume that the rest of the errors, about 23.3 per cent, did not cause any harm according to this study.

The percentage of medical errors attributed to negligence increased in the categories of more severe injuries. Rates of errors rose with the age of the patient, and the percentage of errors due to negligence was markedly higher among the elderly. There were significant differences in rates of errors among categories of *clinical specialties* but with no differences in the percentage due to negligence.

The conclusion from this study was that there was substantial amount of injury to hospital patients from medical management and many injuries were potentially preventable. Rates of errors increased with age, elderly patients being at a higher risk of an adverse event. There was no difference in the incidence of errors among the sexes with regard to negligence. There were variations among specialties for errors but not those due to negligence.

References

1. Laurent Degos and colleagues, Breaking the Mould in Patient Safety, *British Medical Journal*, 2009, **339**, 82-5.
2. Soop et al., The Incidence of Adverse Events in Swedish Hospitals: A Retrospective Record Review Study, *International Journal for Quality in Health Care*, 2009, **21**, 285-91.
3. Rebecca Smith, Thousands of NHS Patients Suffer Avoidable Medical Errors Says Health Commission Annual Report (2008), *Telegraph*, 10 December, 2008, *http://www.telegraph.co.uk/health/3702222*
4. Sari et al., Extent, Nature, and Consequences of Adverse Events: Results of a Retrospective Case Note Review in a Large NHS Hospital, *Qual. Safe Health Care*, 2007, **16**, 434-7.
5. Emily Cook, Women at Risk as 200 Epidural Injections Are Botched a Year, *Daily Mail*, UK, 19 June, 2006.
6. Leape and Berwick, Five Years After 'To Err is Human', What Have We Learned? *Journal of the American Medical Association*, 2005, **293**, 2384-90.
7. Rothschild, Jeffrey M., Landrigan, Christopher P. et al., The Critical Care Safety Study, the incidence and nature of adverse events and serious medical errors in intensive care, *Critical Care Medicine*, 2005, **33**(8), 1694-700.
8. Adams and Boscarino, A Community Survey of Medical Errors in New York, *Int. J. Qual. Health Care*, 2004, 13, ii52-6.
9. Nicola Woolcock and Mark Henderson, Blundering Hospitals 'Kill' 40,000 Every Year, *The Times* (UK), No. 68153, 14 August, 2004, *www.timesonline.co.uk*
10. Dr Foster, CRUK Mortality figures, *British Medical Journal*, 2004, **329**, 369.
11. Sarah Boseley, Medical Errors 'Common' in NHS, *The Guardian*, 6 May, 2003, 5.
12. Angela Coulter, After Bristol: Putting Patients at Centre, *British Medical Journal*, 2002, **324**, 648-51.
13. Robert. L. Poole, William. E. Benitz, et al., Medical Errors in Children, *Journal of the American Medical Association*, 2001, **286**(8), 915-6.
14. Robert. L. Poole, William. E. Benitz, et al., *Journal of the American Medical Association*, 2001, **285**(16), 2141-2.

15. Weingart, S. N., Wilson, R. M. et al., Epidemiology of Medical Error, *British Medical Journal*, 2000, **320**(7237), 774-7, *http:// en,wikipedia.org/wiki/Medical-error*

16. Gaba D., Anesthesiology as a Model for Patient Safety in Health Care, *British Medical Journal*, 2000, **320**, 785-8.

17. Christopher M. Hughes et al., Institute of Medicine (IOM): How Many Deaths are Due to Medical Errors? *Journal of the American Medical Association*, 2000, **284**(17), 2187.

18. Clement. J. McDonald, Michael Weiner, Sui L. Hui, Deaths Due to Medical Errors Are Exaggerated in Institute of Medicine Report, *Journal of the American Medical Association*, 2000, **284**(1), 93-5.

19. Lucian L. Leape, Institute of Medicine Medical Error Figures Are Not Exaggerated, *Journal of the American Medical Association,* 2000, **284**(1), 95-7.

20. Jane Smith, Study into Medical Errors Planned for UK, *British Medical Journal*, 1999, **319**, 1091.

21. Rebecca Voelker, Treat Systems, Not Errors, Experts Say, *Journal of the American Medical Association,* 1996, **276**, 1537-8.

22. Prof. Lucian Leape, Error in Medicine, *Journal of the American Medical Association*, 1994, **272**(23) 1851-7.

23. Prof. Lucian Leape, T. A. Brennam, Nan M. Land, et al., Incidence of Adverse Events and Negligence in Hospitalized Patients, *The New England Journal of Medicine*, 1991, **324**, 370-6.

Chapter 5

Underlying causal factors in the occurrence of Medical Errors and Adverse Events

Human Factors and Ergonomics

The culture of doctors not admitting their problems is changing. All doctors' training is geared towards the other people, that is, their patients, frequently to the detriment of the doctors' psychological and physical health. Doctors have to cope with ever-increasing expectations from patients, and many in practice today, who joined the profession a decade or two ago, now find themselves doing a completely different job to the one they started with. There is decreased job satisfaction and increased anxiety and depression in both hospital and general practice doctors. There is a higher risk of suicide among doctors compared to the general population as confirmed by the Oxford Study (UK) covering the 1957-83 period.

Another large-scale study, based on data obtained from two samples of over eleven thousand respondents in the National Health Service (NHS) workforce, was carried out between 1996 and 1998.

The *first* sample was collected over the 1994 to 1996 period (1996 sample) and the *second* was done over the 1996 to 1998 period(1998 sample). The study examined levels of *stress* amongst *employees* in the NHS trusts, work factors associated with stress, the relationship of stress with sickness, absence, and the effectiveness of selected interventions in reducing stress at the workplace. The principle measure of stress used in the study was the General Health Questionnaire (GHQ-12; Goldberg 1972 and Goldberg and Williams 1991), which was developed as a self-administered screening test for minor psychiatric disorders in the general population. It was chosen because it was one of the best established short instruments available and had been widely used in both community and workplace studies, thus allowing comparisons.

The overall percentage of people suffering from significant levels of stress was 26.8 per cent in the 1996 study group and 26.6 per cent in the 1998 study group. For doctors, the percentages were 27.8 per cent (1996 study group) and 24.6 per cent (1998 study group). The small but notable decrease in numbers of stressed doctors in the 1998 study group was attributed to the reduction in working hours of junior doctors during that period.

Stress is an intrinsic part of medical practice and is encountered every day by doctors. It is a major contributing factor in the occurrence of medical errors. It impairs doctors who are vulnerable, making them unable to practice safely and competently. Many factors are involved in the cause of stress. The pace of new developments in medicine, increased patient expectations, and the fear of litigation are but a few. Errors increase under stress, but stress is not all bad. A little anxiety improves performance, and performance is best at moderate levels of arousal. The improved performance, normally through adaptations, is however short-lived and is soon followed by poor quality performance and uneconomical health care. Poor performance occurs at both extremes—*boredom* and *panic*. Stress is directly related to the job specifications and working conditions, the relationship with people at the workplace, or to a combination of both of these. Conflicts with managers or subordinates and other colleagues may increase under stress as work becomes more pressured. Mental and emotional strain has increased in the new working environments that are characterised by lack of time, more uncontrollable factors, lots of background distractions, lack of space, general uncertainty, and more administrative work.

The *causes of stress*, therefore, are complex but research has pointed to the following factors:

Sleep deprivation in quality and quantity leads to a decrease in mood and performance. Overall evidence suggests that sleep deprivation impairs the doctor's cognitive processing, although in more realistic situations, motivation can compensate for the decreased ability with increased effort and arousal. Effects are greatest upon vigilance-dependent tasks in which infrequent stimuli are detected in a monotonous, uniform environment. Good communication, essential for good caring, depends on the mood of the doctor. Sleep-deprived doctors suffer dysphoric mood changes, including increased anger, hostility, and sadness, decreased elation, decreased affection, and vigour. Affected doctors may communicate less well, especially when things have gone wrong. In a profession like medicine, which is *unforgiving of minor slips*, sleep deprivation is believed to seriously impair clinical performance and judgement. A British judge, Lord Rea, linked doctors' long working hours to medical malpractice claims, and soon after that, a government bill limiting doctors' working hours was introduced in 1989, and it became law soon afterwards. We now have in place the European Working Time Directive. Previously an American court, in 1988, had ruled that long working hours of a hospital resident (doctor) contributed to the death of a patient, known as Libby Zion.

Extreme demands of the working environment may include long working hours under the same environment, high responsibility, and commitment. Long working hours interfere with sleep, the consequences of which have already been discussed.

Organizational culture, which does not allow for weakness, uncertainty, and lack of control, produces a breed of doctors permanently stressed.

Repetitive tasks lead to boredom and are common in medical practice; *boredom*, like *panic*, does produce stress.

Alcohol and drug abuse may follow stress and may lead to more problems and higher risks of making errors.

The General Adaptation Syndrome (GAS) described by the psychologist Seyle, in 1975, characterises the process of prolonged exposure to stress and is a useful staged concept as discussed next.

The alarm reaction stage (or phase): This is the initial reaction stage when triggers (or stressors) are active. These are agents which trigger the various stress reactions. The prevailing working environment provides physical, emotional, and mental stressors, which set off the initial alarm reaction. Stressors can be additive and build up. A single stressor can also become compounded if elements in the support system fail. The way in which people may be affected by stress depends on their values, experience, and adaptability.

The resistance stage (or phase): This follows long exposure to stressors, and during this stage, people develop a 'survival' strategy and a way of fighting against the response the stressor has initiated. The coping mechanism may or may not be adequate to counteract this phase. People prefer short-term relief to long-term solutions, and they try to escape uncomfortable situations with quick remedies. Unfortunately, most easy and short-term measures are inadequate, because they usually lead to secondary problems such as long-term reduction in performance.

The exhaustion stage (or phase): The stress response may be healthy in origin and necessary to keep a person motivated and adaptable, but when the demands on body and mind are too high or cannot be met in an appropriate way, the person affected becomes *depressed*. Prolonged stress can lead to chronic problems and ultimately to exhaustion of all reserves and energies or even to frank depression. Mental dysfunction in the exhaustion stage presents as lack of concentration and coordination which inevitably leads to impaired performance and judgement as well as indecisiveness and a negative attitude toward work. The deterioration in performance is soon accompanied by the occurrence of errors.

Intrinsic stress in the medical profession, in particular, results from one or more of the following situations peculiar to medicine:

a)   *Working with intensely emotional aspects of life* governed by strong cultural codes of behaviour: The examples here are *suffering, fear, sexuality,* and *death*.

Suffering: Doctors' chosen careers consist of routinely interacting with people who are anxious, uncomfortable, and often unable to express gratitude or affection. Doctors are not expected to judge patients who are in a state called *illness*. The acutely ill problem-patient may be a *social paragon*, i.e., a model of excellence, after discharge from hospital. Patients expect more sympathy and skill in relieving their symptoms than most modern doctors can provide. Modern doctors are also hampered by poor communication with their patients. They rely on fallible institutions. Repeated contact with their patients could enhance the accuracy of intuitive judgements. Pain descriptions may elicit suspicion rather than the compassion expected by their patients, usually due to fear of manipulation by patients with drug-acquisitive behaviour. The doctor is entrusted, not only with the relief of pain, but also with decisions to inflict pain, prescribe pressures, or deny the palliative treatment of discomfort. Occasions to inflict pain or deny palliation have multiplied with the increase in opportunities to make precise diagnosis and sophisticated in vivo measurements and to sustain vegetative functions.

Fear. The primary and ultimate reason for consulting a doctor by a patient is fear. Calm, relaxed behaviour is uncommon enough for a physician to suspect abnormal patient behaviour. Fearful patients are fatiguing and unpleasant to work with. Fear is often contagious, especially if the doctor gets personally involved or identifies with the patient's problems. Doctors should avoid such involvement by skilful treatment of the illness and by reassurance given to their patients.

Sexuality: A doctor is entitled and is required to probe into areas of the body hidden from all others and into the private aspects of a patient's life. The patient may harbour ambivalent feelings about the doctor's privileged role. There is fear that these privileges and powers could be abused. Doctors, too, may be ambivalent. Civilised desire to respect the patient's modesty and avoid the anxiety of emotional and physical nakedness is countered by the obligations that accompany special privileges and responsibilities.

Practising doctors experience embarrassment when caring for friends, family members, or their colleagues. Emotional distancing gets lost, and the desire to preserve modesty conflicts with the need to acquire clinical information. Embarrassment never completely disappears from the act of obtaining clinical history and performing a physical examination. Demands for careful data collection should not be ignored because of the guilty feelings on the part of the physician.

Death: Death is usually seen by the patient's family and by some doctors as a failure of medical care. Most doctors work in the fear of or in the presence of death of the patient, and familiarity does not remove its sting. Communication between the patient, the patient's family, and the doctor frequently breaks down when the patient is dying. Dying is a major social issue, and nobody is comfortable talking about the realities of death. Even the very informed, well-consulted family members may turn against the doctor in anger when the patient dies. In today's technological advances where patients are put on life support systems, the doctor is placed in the absurdly stressful situation of *killing* the patient by discontinuing the use of the life support equipment and drug therapy!

b) *Inadequate training for fundamental professional tasks,* like handling *problem-patients,* creates a common problem to doctors. Stereotypes of *clingers* and *demanders, help-rejectors* and *deniers* are familiar to all doctors. They elicit anger, avoidance, fear, and despair. These patients cannot and will not get better. Most of them have important or significant psychiatric disorders which underlie their frustrating interactions with doctors.

Doctors rarely know or acquire the techniques needed to take care of this type of patients. Problem-patients seek medical care much more often than the ordinary patients do, and many of these even constitute a large percentage of clinical patients. The amount of time spent by primary care doctors in caring for problem-patients has increased very dramatically over the last few decades. There is need for a more proactive process to help doctors cope with stress generated by these patients. Training doctors in stress management should highlight this part of modern medical practice.

c) *Demands from society and patients* that cannot reasonably be met under current medical knowledge, which only allows for approximation, is yet another factor in the prevalence of intrinsic stress among doctors. Medical training consists of learning to cope with pervasive uncertainty within the limits of medical knowledge. Balancing the demands of patients for definitive diagnosis with those of health-care planners for cost-effective use of limited resources can make the diagnosis and treatment of even the 'trivial' a bewildering series of uncertain decisions. The stress of uncertainty tempts both the patient and the doctor to *collude* in oversimplifications and *lies.* Falsehoods, however, break down communication and bring new moral and emotional consequences for the doctor. Common adaptation, which is developing standard clinical routines or habits, may reduce the stress of making decisions, but it can increase the cost of medical care with little or no clinical benefit. Furthermore, both the patient and the doctor are often uncomfortable today in what seemed to be or was a stable, predictable relationship.

Patients reward doctors who conform to their perceptions about how doctors should look and behave. Doctors who happen to be of the *wrong* sex or race or those who dress unconventionally will have problematic encounters with some types of patients and their families. Demands for conformity to social conventions for behaviour and appearance also have profound effect on the doctor's personal as well as family life.

d) *Information in medical practice* lacks the structure needed to efficiently connect those who produce and achieve medical knowledge to those who must apply that knowledge. There are serious 'voltage drops' along the transmission line for medical knowledge in the current health-care system. This means only a proportion of medical knowledge is ever loaded into the minds of professionals. Not all knowledge so loaded is retained, and much of the knowledge so retained becomes obsolete. There is no assurance that the professionals will learn new knowledge relevant to their patients' problems. Even with the limited knowledge retained, doctors' minds cannot reliably integrate that knowledge with the infinite variety of data about patients in order to identify and systematically assess all diagnostic and treatment options based on each patient's unique characteristics and needs. Faced with information overload, doctors fall back on 'clinical judgement', which is a global intuitive assessment of findings rather than organised investigation and explicit linkage of each finding in the patient to the relevant diagnostic and management options in medical literature. Cognitive psychology shows that experts' global judgements are inferior to judgements based on thorough analysis of specific data.

Doctors not only rely improperly on their global judgements but also habitually fail to gather or consider information relevant to their judgements. This happens because graduate medical 'education' instils into them a faith that they can safely rely on the limited information their minds can process, such faith being a necessary defence mechanism for the unaided mind and also because medical education and practice reward specialisation. Specialisation does allow a lot of exclusions in medical education and practice. The unaided mind's normal functioning uses techniques most suited for discarding information. Cognitive pitfalls and textbook classifications of diseases cause doctors to focus on the few known characteristics that a patient shares with others who have the 'same diagnosis' while discounting the hundreds of characteristics that make the patient different from those others and may have more to do with the patient's therapeutic needs than the diagnostic label.

For financial and demographic reasons, many people who need medical care have little or no access to the medical knowledge residing in expensively educated geographically limited doctors. Nor do they have sufficient access to the skills that doctors possess, because the rules of accreditation mean that the same professional group monopolises both skills and knowledge. Good medical practice requires means to extend the human mind's limited capacity to recall and process large numbers of relevant variables. Today, knowledge is also held in computers and other machinery, from where it is used routinely and kept up to date relatively cheaply. This approach has allowed a defined and consistent mechanism of controlling and keeping track of inputs to the health-care system, which in turn, enables outputs to be properly interpreted and corrective feedback loops to be used routinely.

The British Medical Association (BMA) has a stress counselling service with a helpline manned by non-medical counsellors. The telephone number is: 0645 200169.

The Association of Anaesthetists of Great Britain and Ireland, *Sick Doctor* scheme operates its own helpline. The telephone number is: 0207 6311650.

References

1. Hanuscak, et al., Evaluation of Causes and Frequency of Medication Errors During Information Technology Downtime, *American Journal of Health-System Pharmacy,* 2009, **66**, 1119-24.
2. Fahrebkopf A. M., et al., Rates of Medication Errors Among Depressed and Burnt-Out Residents: Prospective Cohort Study, *British Medical Journal,* 2008, **336**(7642), 488-91. *www.bmj.com/cgi/content/full/bmj39469*
3. Landrigan, et al., Effects of Accreditation Council for Graduate Medical Education Duty Hour Limits, Sleep, Work Hours and Safety, *Pediatrics,* 2008, **122**, 250-8.
4. Editor (Incidence of stress), *Occupational Health Statistics Bulletin* 2004/5, *www.hse.gov.uk/statistics/overall/ohsb0405.htm*

5. Department of Health (DoH): Improving Working Lives for Doctors, *Department of Health* Booklet, *www.doh.gov.uk/iwl/2004*

6. Editor (20 Tips to Prevent Medical Errors), *www.ahrg.gov/consumer/20tips.htm*

7. Editor (Tired, Stressed doctors), *www.news.bbc.co.uk/2/hi/health/4080424*

8. Editor (Perceived Stress, Sources, and Severity of Stress Among Medical Doctors, *www.ukpmc.ac.uk/abstract/MED/20078853*

9. Editor (Stress and Work), *www.agius.com/hew/resource/stress.htm*

10. National Academy of Sciences, To Err Is Human, The National Academies Press, 2000, *www.nap.edu/catalog.php/record-id-9728*

11. Weingart, Saul, et al., Epidemiology of Medical Error, *British Medical Journal*, 2000, **320**(7237), 774-7.

12. Nocera A. Khursandi, Doctors Working Hours: Can the Medical Profession Afford to Let the Courts Decide What Is Reasonable? *Medical Journal of Australia*, 1998, **168**(12), 616-8, *www.mja.com.au/public/issues/june15/nocera.html*

13. Paul Dinsdale, Doctors Are Top of the Stress League, *Hospital Doctor* (UK), 19 November, 1998, 17.

14. Lawrence L. Weed, New Connections Between Medical Knowledge and Patient Care, *British Medical Journal*, 1997, **315**, 231-5.

15. Prof. Carlo Fonseka, To Err Was Fatal, *British Medical Journal*, 1996, **313**, 1640-2.

16. Julia von Onciul, Stress at Work, *British Medical Journal*, 1996, **313**, 745-8.

17. H. F. Seeley, The Practice of Anaesthesia; A Stressor for Middle-aged? *Anaesthesia*, 1996, **51**, 571-4.

18. C. A. Vincent, Research into Medical Accidents; A Case of Negligence? *British Medical Journal*, 1989, **299**, 1150-3.

19. R. A. J. Asher, The Dangers of Not Going to Bed, *The Lancet*, 1989, 138-9.

20. Jack. D. McCue, The Effects of Stress on Physicians and Their Medical Practice,

21. *The New England Journal of Medicine*, 1982, **306**(8) 458-63.

Chapter 6

Common Causes of Medical Errors

Human error is still the most common cause of medical errors. J. Cooper et al, in a study done in 1978, found that *82 per cent* of medical errors were due to human error. Some of the causal factors in human error identified in that study included the following:

Fatigue; distraction or inattention and carelessness; visual restrictions; inadequate familiarity with the equipment; inadequate training; inadequate supervision; inexperience of the doctor; and poor doctor-patient communication.

Exchange of personnel during procedures was another factor, but the authors were of the view that the policy which encouraged relief of personnel was much preferred to one that did not.

In this study, it was also found that *12 per cent* of errors were due to *equipment failure* and a smaller percentage was due to complicated or poorly designed equipments.

The inherent uncertainty of medical practice creates a situation in which errors are always possible. Each of myriad decisions made every day has the potential for drastic consequences if it is not determined properly. It is highly likely that sooner or later, doctors will make mistakes that seriously harm or are fatal to their patients. The drastic consequences of the doctors' errors, the repeated opportunities to make errors, the uncertainty about the doctors' culpability when results are poor, and the medical and social denial that errors must happen all result in an intolerable paradox for doctors.

There is no absolute certainty in medical science. Scientific knowledge is conjectural and hypothetical. Old ethics lead to intellectual dishonesty by upholding the idea of authority. *Authority* tends to become important in its own right. An authority is not expected to err, and when errors occur, they tend to be covered up to uphold the idea of authority. Thus, the old ethics lead doctors to hide their errors, and the consequences were worse than the errors hidden. Old ethics influenced the medical education system, which encouraged the accumulation of knowledge and its 'regurgitation' in examinations. Students were punished for their mistakes, and they, therefore, hid them from their peers. This made correction of students' deficiencies very difficult. Since then, a new professional code of training and practice has emerged with notable improvement in error prevention and management.

Medical errors and adverse events are a result of the interaction of patients, patients' diseases, and a complicated highly technical system of medical care providers, *not only* a diverse group of doctors, other health-care providers and support personnel, *but also* a medical industrial system that supplies the drugs and equipments. Causes of medical errors, therefore, can be multiple-determined and it can be difficult to identify a single overriding cause.

Causal factors underlying medical errors include the following:

Medical advances—all high risk specialties face twin challenges. Technical and medical advances mean more can be attempted, but the expectations of the public is of a total cure for every illness, with decreasing tolerance of any failure to cure. High expectations often lead to family anger and a search for reprisal. There is need for a change in the culture of distrust and the equation of any complication or poor outcome with negligence.

Personal characteristics—may play a part in the occurrence of errors. However, there is no proven accident-prone personality. Some individuals make more mistakes than others at particular times and under particular circumstances. High anxiety levels, depression, overconfidence, willingness to make risky decisions, and basic clinical incompetence may predispose one to making errors in clinical practice.

Transient stages may be due to the effects of drugs and alcohol. Their role in the occurrence of medical errors is unquantified. Fatigue and mood swings need further investigation.

Patient characteristics can influence the occurrence of errors. The patients' combination of signs and symptoms and the history of his illness may increase the liability to err. Factors affecting communication between the doctor and patient may also be contributory to error occurrence. Diagnostic errors may result from doctor and patient language difficulties which compromise reliable communication.

Organizational factors are implicated in some medical accidents. Poor staffing levels lead to overwork and fatigue. Shift patterns, workload, and several tasks done at once do increase the risk of errors. Administrative efficacy may influence the availability of patients' records, test results, and the ease of communication between team members as well as the accessibility of necessary staff.

Complexity of the disease and treatments plays a major part in the occurrence of errors in hospitalised patients. Special medical conditions involve the choice of a variety of drugs, sometimes given over very long periods of treatment. So it is not surprising that quality and the variety of drugs administered influence error occurrence, mainly from drug interactions, drug side effects, routes of administration, and wrong dosages.

The age of the patient is yet another important factor. It has been known for a long time that elderly patients do have a high risk of being involved in adverse medical events. These patients are more likely not only to have more complicated diseases, but also to have underlying degenerative conditions which increase the risk of such non-technical complications as myocardial infarcts, pulmonary emboli, congestive cardiac failure, cerebral vascular accidents, and pneumonia. Errors which are well tolerated by children and young, healthy adults can be fatal in the elderly and in those patients weakened by disease or those with impaired vital organs.

Medical nature and frequency of interactions are important factors. Conditions under which doctors in some specialties work are far less forgiving than others. Interventions from specialties such as neurosurgery, obstetrics, thoracic and vascular surgery and anaesthesia and intensive care may generate not only adverse incidents, but much more serious such incidents. In a typical hospitalisation, a patient may have hundreds of encounters with doctors, nurses, and other hospital staff, all employing various medical equipments. Every medical intervention carries with it some level of risk.

Location where medical care is provided may have an influence on the occurrence of errors and adverse events. **Accident and Emergency Units (A and E Units)** and **Intensive Care Units (ICUs)**, **High Dependence Units**, and **Operating Theatres** are places in a hospital where medical errors, and especially the more serious ones, are more likely to occur. Doctors in A and E Units have less time to spend with each patient because of the volume of work and changing priorities in their workplace. The ICU is usually inhabited by very sick, high-risk patients undergoing multiple and complex interventions.

System failure: Humans make up a system which is run by humans. The vast majority of errors are due to system failure rather than negligence or incompetence of the doctors. The need, therefore, is to treat the system rather than the error. Here in the UK, general practitioners (GPs) have in the past tended to suffer from poor organisation, poor follow-up of their patients, and a failure to apply consistent criteria for diagnosis and treatment of patients. Changes to their contracts, continuing professional development seminars, and introduction of tighter General Medical Council regulation and supervision have led to very significant improvement in their services and a reduction in the risk to err. Hospital doctors, on the other hand, usually have smaller numbers of errors, probably because of the better organization, better follow-up regimes, higher alert due to the seriousness of hospital patients' illnesses, and better facilities to diagnose, monitor, and treat their patients. Hospital doctors also have more support staff at their disposal.

Doctor-patient communication: Never before has the *need* for *good communication* in health care been more acute. How and what doctors and nurses speak to their patients is the most important aspect of communication. Effective communication enables patients to make decisions about their care and to make choices about alternative treatments. Effective communication is the doctor's moral obligation and responsibility to his/her patients. There is a great deal of questioning about how doctors communicate with their patients and about their perceived unwillingness to communicate to their patients *poor practice* when they know about it. Improved interaction between doctors, other medical professionals, and their patients should come about by introducing a greater element of joint training in ethical issues and communication skills.

Communication delivery is 7 per cent by *words* used, 38 per cent by the *tone of the voice,* and 55 per cent by the *body language,* according to one study. The doctor who sits beside the patient is offering to share control of the situation. Non-verbal communication is a crucial part of the process of establishing a rapport between doctor and patient. Patients want attention lavished on their problems, but unfortunately, doctors are under pressure and rushed off their feet. One solution has been to improve doctor's language. Non-verbal signs can be as important as verbal, and using them effectively can save doctors a lot of trouble in the long run. What is said may be less important than how it is said. What is left unsaid and interpreted from coded messages constitute body language. But there is a word of caution; body language is a complex means of communication and can be very confusing both to the doctor and patient, particularly if practiced by people from different cultural backgrounds. The hospital environment makes patients nervous and worried. Doctors are on home ground, have status, prestige, and power by virtue of their position. The least patients expect is a proper greeting and a smile, which is a sign of sympathy and warmth, not amusement. Doctors should not carry the 'graveyard look' with them and should not copy the patients' look of worry and anxiety.

Doctors should show that they are listening and listening well. Good eye contact indicates good attention in Western cultures, and a smile shows sympathy. An open posture shows an open mind while crossing legs shows defensiveness and closure. A worried patient may initially adopt this posture but during a meaningful conversation, it is natural for one to mimic the position of the other. Doctors should maintain an open posture and wait for the patient to adopt a similar posture as he/she relaxes. In spite of the previous word of *caution,* it is worth remembering that most body languages cross ethnic, national, and gender barriers. Greetings share common elements of smiling, eye contact, and open palms. Doctors who pay attention to the multilayered messages contained within body language will not only improve the quality of their diagnosis but also help make their patients' experiences of a hospital visit less unpleasant.

References

1. Wikipedia, Medical Error, *http://en.wikipedia.org/wiki/Medicalerrors/2000*

2. Medical Errors and Patient Safety, *www.ahrg.gov/qual/errorsix.htm, www.ahcpr.gov/qual/errorsix.htm*

3. Medical Errors Kill Tens of Thousands Annually, *www.cnn.com/HEALTH/99911/29/medical.errors.*

4. Report to the President (USA) on Medical Errors, *www.quic.gov/report*

5. Benjamin. W. Lamb and Kamal Nagpal, Importance of Near Misses, *British Medical Journal*, 2009, **339**, 255.

6. Nicola Woolcock, Elderly Men Most at Risk of Hospital Error, *The Times*, 13 August, 2004, 4.

7. Neale. G., et al., Exploring the Causes of Adverse Events in NHS Hospital Practice, *Journal of Royal Society of Medicine*, 2001, **94**(7), 322-30.

8. Reason. J. T., Human Error, Models and Management, *British Medical Journal*, 2000, **320**, 768-70.

Chapter 7

Informed Consent: Other Theories of Consent and their relevance to Medical Errors and Adverse Events

Thomas Percival, in his book *Medical Ethics* published in 1803, argued that 'to a patient who makes inquiries which, if truthfully answered, might prove fatal to him, it would be a gross and unfeeling wrong to tell the truth.' Nearly fifty years later, in the 1850s, Worthington Hooker of Connecticut, USA, took issue with Percival in his book, *Physician and Patient*, but his arguments had little impact with the medical profession of the time. Similar pleas by D. W. Cathell, in 1885, and Austin Flint in 1898, were also largely ignored. Reverend Russel Dicks, in the 1930s, in collaboration with Dr Richard Cabot, wrote a chapter entitled 'The Dying', part of a book entitled *The Art of Ministering to the Sick*. Reverend Russel Dicks did admit to having learnt openness from the seriously ill and made reference to the heroism of the dying and to the privilege of having shared in their extremity. At about the same time, Lawrence Henderson, a brilliant chemist, gave a Harvard University address entitled *Physician and Patient as a Social System* at the end of which he said and I quote, ' . . . try to modify the patient's sentiments to his own advantage and remember that nothing is more effective than arousing the belief that you are concerned wholeheartedly and exclusively for his welfare'.

In 1950, Dean Willard Sperry of Harvard Divinity School, USA, deplored the outspokenness of his physician colleagues. He concluded that whether the physician is to tell the truth depends primarily on his knowledge of the patient and the patient's frame of mind. Today, a majority of doctors have gone from *not telling* to *telling*. Doctors, wisely enough, cannot decide in advance which patient should or should not be told the truth. They can, however, sense which of their patients would be difficult to tell. Shielding is ultimately impossible, and the price of its temporary achievement is an enduring sense of betrayal. *Lying* is wrong, but there are possible exceptions when dealing with medical information and decisions. Doctors need to look further into themselves and ask why they falter at telling bad news or manage its consequences badly—how often it is a blinking at their own mortality, a reluctance to admit the failure of what they have done for prevention or cure, or unworthy desire to control.

Theories of Consent

Consent is understood differently by various disciplines and professions and there are various theoretical models. These models are discussed as follows:

Real Consent: Positivist surveys dominate research about consent. They mainly measure information given. Problems in real consent are attributed to patients' and doctors' limited knowledge and communication skills and are addressed by efforts to improve knowledge and skill. Social pressures and great anxiety and distress are assumed to inhibit patients' ability to make independent, rational choices and so should be reduced or avoided where possible. The respect for informed consent within a positive framework brings important benefits, some of which are to encourage professionals in health care to be accountable and to know and explain clearly what they plan to do and why. Basic information standards are agreed and are achieved partly through research, audit, and professional education.

Respect for patients' consent or refusal provides recognition for their physical and mental integrity. It defends patients from un-consented interventions and from deception or coercion during treatment or research. However, positivist theories set such high standards that many people are classified as ignorant, too dependent, or too emotional to be competent. Because real consent is unrealistic for many ordinary people, clinicians and researchers feel cynical, irritated, or despondent about it.

Constructed Consent: Modern ideas of consent began in the seventeenth century and are used in varying and contradictory ways. The two main components of modern consent are *understanding* and *voluntariness*. These originate from seventeenth century religious beliefs that intellect and will are the two things that make us human. Thus, theories of consent are based on personal and social beliefs about human nature. Consent is integral to modern democracy, which was also born at that time as the idea that we have enough understanding and will withdraw consent from inadequate rulers. Consent, then, was seen largely as an act of the will. Professional assessments of adequate information and competence to consent can be seen as varying social constructs, not universal standards.

Positivism tends to see patients' abilities as fixed personal attributes. Social construction sees patients' abilities partly as responses in relations influenced by the professionals' abilities to explain, respect, and support. In real consent, all influences tend to be seen as potentially coercive pressures and autonomy is seen as free-floating individualism. Social construction shows how we would not have choices or ability to choose between them. Relationships can enrich as well as restrict the autonomy to consent.

Functional Consent: Functionalist consent is a polite ceremony, a token of respect that is hardly necessary because benign expert doctors contribute to the smooth functioning of society; refusal and non-compliance is irrational. Consent is, however, a convenient means of transferring responsibility for risk from the doctor or researcher to the informed patient, thus enabling treatment and research to proceed without serious risk of costly litigations. Most people are partly functionalists in that they need to be members of a coherent society with some consensus on stable useful knowledge. Many doctors would not explicitly support extreme functionalism, but in a busy workplace like wards, clinics, and surgeries, consent tended to be treated as a simple tedious formality.

Critical Theory: There is a view which sees consent as necessary protection for patients against useless, harmful, and unwanted interventions, an occasion when doctors have to be accountable. It is, to them, an essential constraint on the most powerful profession. Informed consent is an exchange of knowledge between doctor and patient so that together they can make more informed decisions.

Postmodernism and Postmodern Choice

In postmodern societies, people have become consumers whose highest value is choice. Political consumers campaign for ethical care and fair rationing; green consumers are keen on keeping fit and on products that are not derived from animal experiments. Consumers, as explorers, go in for exotic treatments. Hedonists consume for pleasure, glamour, and attention, and are seen in advertisements for private health insurance and health reforms. All this may seem a travesty of real consent and serious medicine, yet postmodernism contributes important insights. Social and economic forces ensure that everyone in wealthy societies is a consumer who expects to be offered choices, best of all, when they are ill or injured.

Informed Consent and Its Relevance to Medical Errors and Adverse Events

Informed consent is defined as 'the voluntary and continuing permission of the patient to receive a particular treatment based on an adequate knowledge of the purpose, nature, likely effects, and risk of that treatment, including the likelihood of its success, alternatives to it, and the likely consequences of refusing that particular treatment'.

Another definition is 'a voluntary un-coerced decision made by a sufficiently competent or autonomous person on the basis of adequate information and deliberation, to accept rather than reject some proposed course of action that will affect him/her'.

Consent to treatment is an essential part of the contract of trust between patient and doctor. Patients, and in the case of children, their parents or guardians, have a right to be fully involved in decisions about their care. For that reason, doctors must do their best to explain to patients the treatments which are proposed and to obtain their patients' informed consent. Informed consent is usually a one-time affair with an operation pending, with its abrupt change of circumstances, usually a general anaesthetic, and until recently, several days of pain and medication afterwards, all ideally suited to resist easy imprinting and to erase any imprinting that may occur. One session may not be enough, and seeking informed consent should not be a one-off affair. It should be a continuing process of open and helpful dialogue integral to the patient's treatment. The doctor should tell all he/she knows as appropriate with a minimum of labels and an absence of jargon and with a conscious effort at transparency to encourage a response in kind. The doctor should not tell more than he/she knows. Admission of ignorance serves to confirm the doctor's knowledge.

The patient or a family member may ask the doctor to peer into the future, and if there is a good reason, the doctor may wish to guess, extrapolate from what has gone on, or invoke prior experience or accept the challenge of doctor so and so. The doctor should resist at least until the patient has reached the narrow place near the end. Trouble can come from more directions than can be predicted, and its timing is its own. Matter-of-factness is crucial. Pity and sympathy are distancing. They separate giver from receiver by emphasising the differences in their lots. People in desperate trouble need sharing, which they get from the acknowledgement in the doctor's words of what they are up against, the promise in the doctor's attentiveness that he/she will be there, and the declaration in his/her attitude that he/she and the patient are fellow wayfarers on a road beset by fate and ending always in the betrayal of the physical self. Most important for the doctor is to keep the patient in charge of his/her destiny.

Consent can or may be Expressed or Implied

Expressed Consent is given when a patient confirms his/her agreement to treatment or procedure in clear or explicit terms, whether orally or in writing. Expressed written consent should be obtained for any procedure or treatment carrying any substantial side effects, including all patients undergoing a procedure under a general anaesthetic. Consent should never be obtained from a patient who has had medication (usually a pre-medication) which impairs his/her judgement. Refusal of part of the procedure or treatment, e.g. blood transfusion, should be specified. A patient does not have the right to demand a particular kind of treatment. Consent from adult patients' next of kin is not valid in the UK. Consent should be obtained from a patient if the proposed treatment or procedure is to be carried out by a health-care professional undergoing training.

Implied Consent is assumed where a patient freely agrees to and complies with a request from a doctor or such health-care professional. Consent is implied if, for example, a patient freely offers an arm to a health-care professional to take a blood sample.

Informed Consent and Minors

In the UK, children under sixteen years of age have the right to give consent provided they have sufficient understanding of the information they are given. Ideally, the parent(s) should also give consent and must always do so if the child does not have sufficient understanding. Between the ages of sixteen and eighteen years, the patient would normally give consent independently. However, parents or guardians may still give consent up to the age of eighteen years if the patient is not competent. In the event of a refusal of parental consent for urgent treatment where it is not feasible to obtain a court order, the procedure should be consented to by two consultants after explaining the risks of withholding such treatment to the patient/parent. A witnessed record of the conversation should be entered in the patient's medical records.

Treatment without the Patient's Consent

The following is a summary of special circumstances under which treatment may have to be administered without the consent of the patient or legal guardian in the UK.

1. *Life saving emergency treatment*: This is treatment carried out to save the patient's life or to prevent other serious harm to the patient or where the patient is unconscious and unable to express his/her wishes.
2. *Where a statutory power exists* requiring the examination of the patient, for example, under regulations governing disease control: An explanation should be provided and consent should be sought in the normal way initially.
3. A *minor* who is a *ward of court* in the UK: A court may decide that treatment is in the best interests of the patient and grants a court order to that effect.
4. *Treatment for a mental disorder* in a patient detained (or sectioned) under the Mental Health Act 1983 of the UK.
5. *Treatment for a physical disorder* when a patient is incapable of giving informed consent by reason of a mental disorder and the treatment is in the patient's best interests.

Timing of Consent: Consent should be obtained long before the proposed procedure is carried out for elective procedures or surgery. This gives the patient the very important 'cooling off' period. However, if the patient's condition alters during this period or if such period is over six months (UK), another consent will be necessary.

The General Medical Council (UK) endorsed the concept of the advance directive or *living will* and advised doctors to respect decisions on refusing treatment made by patients before they have lost the capacity to do so. A 'living will' should be verified and be part of the patient's medical records.

The General Medical Council (GMC) and Consent: The General Medical Council approved a set of guidelines giving the treating doctor explicit responsibility for obtaining 'informed consent' from the patient unless this is not practicable. Consent for elective procedures should be obtained by a doctor who is competent in explaining the risks and benefits of the proposed treatment as well as being capable of performing such a procedure the patient is to undergo. The GMC booklet entitled, *Seeking Patients' Consent; the Ethical Considerations* contains guidelines on issues doctors should consider before, during, and after obtaining patients' consent to investigations, treatment, screening, and research. It stresses the fact that it is for the patient, not the doctor, to make the final decision. It also explains how to get consent in an emergency and from patients whose capabilities to make decisions are impaired. It covers consent for *clinical trials* as well.

Informed Consent and Research: Research, including clinical research, is aimed, not only at the good of the individual patient or participant, but also at the production of medical knowledge which is for the good of society at large. This is the difference between research and the use of innovative treatment for an individual patient. The moral principle involved here is referred to as the *principle of autonomy or non-exploitation.* Where research involves areas of clinical medicine where disease(s) causing the patient's incompetence to consent are being researched, then it is necessary to resort to *consent by proxy.* Heather Goodare (*British Medical Journal,* 1998, **316**, 1004-5) suggested that research studies that do not have informed consent from participants should not be published. This is now the stated policy of doctors and researchers who observe 'uniform requirements for manuscripts submitted to biomedical journals'. The Nuremberg Code or its watered down form, the Declaration of Helsinki, states that 'the voluntary consent of the human subject is absolutely essential'. The Declaration of Helsinki introduced a section (Clause 11.5) on clinical research which says that 'if a doctor considers it essential not to obtain informed consent, the specific reasons for this proposal should be stated in the experimental protocol for transmission to the independent committee'.

The British Medical Journal (BMJ) changed its policy on consent for publishing materials that emerge from the doctor-patient relationship. It moved to 'informed consent' for all such material, and this is the position adopted by the International Committee of Medical Journal Editors (ICMJE). The General Medical Council adopted the same line.

Publication *without consent* may be acceptable in the following cases:

* Where the patient is long dead and has no living relatives.
* Where the medical interaction took place a long time earlier, perhaps over fifteen years ago, especially where interaction involved the elderly or terminally ill patients.
* If the relevant piece of research is to be published without the names of patients attached, making it difficult or unlikely for anybody to identify the patients.
* Publication without consent may also be acceptable in situations where information has been disguised or fictionalised, but these situations may carry a lot of danger and are not advisable.

Scientific Research fraud: This undermines trust and damages confidence in the medical profession in general and in medical research in particular. It puts patients at risk as it may lead to false and potentially dangerous conclusions, which filter through into clinical practice. The GMC continues to emphasise the need for integrity in research and applies severe sanctions when doctors are found guilty of research-related misconduct. Its guidance on this matter is clear; doctors taking part in clinical trials must record their research results truthfully. Dishonesty or fraudulent record-keeping by doctors participating in research is not only discreditable in itself but also a potential source of danger to patients.

Competition for research funds may compromise the protection of participants. Recruitment of such participants through the *media* is also unfavourable as such advertisements play down the risks of being in an experiment and they emphasise only the potential benefits, such as free health check-ups. The health of participants may not be the primary concern of investigators, and some participants will be in the *placebo group*. Many potential participants, therefore, may not be giving a true 'informed consent'. Knowing about risks is a prerequisite for research participants to exercise their common law right to give informed consent.

Informed Consent, Language, and Religious Barriers

Informed consent and language difficulties or barriers have been ignored for a long time and little addressed at world medical forums. This also applies to informed consent and religious or cultural barriers.

Medical practice should not have barriers, but informed consent should recognise and, where possible, address such barriers. Doctors whose language may not be the first or second language of their patients may get into difficulties when it comes to obtaining informed consent and when interpreting medical findings or instituting treatments. Some *ethnic* and *religious* groups may have different ways of giving consent for certain medical interventions and by which *gender* of the medical practitioner involved. This may influence the outcome of medical interventions. Whereas it is impossible for the medical profession to be fully equipped to deal with these concerns, training of and provision of interpreters should be part of the practice of medicine in an ever-increasing multicultural and religiously diverse society. The role of relatives, next of kin, and religious leaders as well as members of the legal profession should be discussed with patients when obtaining informed consent. National governments should address this problem by incorporating clauses in laws on medical practice which deal with such problems and situations.

Clinical management of a Jehovah's Witness: For a Jehovah's Witness, the prohibition of blood and blood-products transfusion is a deeply held core value and is a sign of respect for life. Some Witnesses may accept plasma protein fraction (PPF) or albumin, immuno-globulins and haemophilic preparations. The Committee of Elders (Hospital Liaison Committee for Jehovah's Witnesses, well established in many cities in the UK) may advise both clinicians and their Jehovah's Witness patients on what is the best course to take if conflicts arise. Most Jehovah's Witnesses carry with them a clear advance directive (*living will*) prohibiting blood transfusions. Such a directive, properly signed and witnessed, must be respected unless there is some reason to suppose that the patient had changed his/her mind since the directive was executed.

Advance Directives ('Living Wills'): These 'wills' are made by competent patients with the intention that they will remain effective if the patients become incompetent. An advance directive may be binding upon clinicians when it expresses a refusal of treatment in circumstances that the patient has anticipated. An advance directive may be ineffective if what ensued was not anticipated by the patient at the time of making it. The clinician should consider very carefully advance directives, bearing in mind the possibility that the patient may have changed his/her mind since signing that advance directive, or other circumstances have occurred and medical science may have developed in unforeseen ways in the interval from signing the directive and the time it becomes operative. For a positive consent to or a claim for certain treatments, clinicians are not legally bound by such consent nor are they compelled to carry out treatments which are contrary to their clinical judgement or those outside of the law. Doctors, however, have a duty to refer these patients to those colleagues willing and able to manage such patients.

The General Medical Council's new guidance on consent, prepared by the GMC's Standards Committee, discusses the ethical issues that doctors should consider before, during, and after obtaining consent from patients for investigations, treatments, screening, and for research. The guideline points out that the amount of information patients are given will vary and the doctors should do their best to find out about patients' individual needs and priorities. Doctors should not make assumptions about patients' views but ask patients whether they have any concerns about the intended treatment or risks involved.

Doctors should not exceed the scope of the authority given by patients, except in an emergency, and they should give clear explanation of the scope of the consent being sought. This is particularly important if different doctors are involved in the patient's care or if there will be several different investigations or treatments. Doctors should not withhold information unless they judge that providing such information would cause the patient serious harm. In cases where doctors decide to withhold information, they must record this fact. In emergencies, doctors may provide treatment limited to what is 'immediately necessary to save life or to avoid significant deterioration in the patient's health'. The GMC warns doctors against relying on a patient's apparent compliance with a procedure as a form of consent, the so called 'implied' consent. For example, the fact that a patient lies down on an examination couch does not in itself indicate that the patient has understood what the doctor proposes to do and why.

Case Reports on Consent in the recent past in the UK

Case 1. A research team that had a radioactive marker injected into patients to help diagnose a neurological disorder was suspected of fabricating their results. There was no evidence that the patients had *consented* to the treatment or that ethical approach had been obtained.

Case 2. A consultant physician was struck off the medical register by the GMC after being found guilty of falsifying patients' key documents in a drug trial. The doctor admitted falsifying patients' *consent forms* and research data in a study on amlodipine.

Case 3. In 1998, a paediatric cardiologist had his registration with the GMC suspended for six months when he carried out a heart procedure on a six-year-old girl without the *consent* of her parents.

Case 4. An enquiry was started in February 1999 into research conducted at the North Staffordshire Hospital (UK) after parents complained that they were misled into *consenting* to experimental treatment for their premature babies. A new type of ventilator was tested between 1989 and 1993 on 122 babies with breathing difficulties in a technique called 'continuous negative extra-thoracic pressure'. Twenty-eight of the babies died and fifteen babies suffered brain damage. Although the difference in results between the test and control groups was thought not to be statistically significant, several families complained that they were unaware of the experimental nature of the treatment. One complainant went as far as claiming that the consent form had been pushed under his nose to sign.

Case 5. In the United Bristol Healthcare NHS Trust, three paediatric consultant cardiologists were involved in certain parents' protests against the removal of their children's hearts and other body tissues. Parents protested over the removal of hearts from their children who had died following heart surgery between 1976 and 1995.

Hearts had been removed systematically, but the trust spokesman said that it was done for the proper examination, education, and for audit purposes as was standard practice in Great Britain at the time. The trust admitted, however, that the *consent* was 'not as informed as modern standards required'. Although consent had been obtained for the normal 'hospital post-mortems' on the children, it was acknowledged that in those days, doctors would not always have fully explained the intricacies of what a post-mortem might entail.

Case 6. In September 1999, a number of consultant cardiologists at the Royal Brompton Hospital, London, were cleared of giving misleading information to patients when obtaining consent. They were also cleared of discriminating against children with Down's syndrome. The report on this case said that the importance of the *consenting process* should be stressed to all relevant medical staff.

Case 7. In November 1999, the British Government launched an independent inquiry into the alleged removal of children's organs without *parental consent* at the Alder Hey Children's Hospital, Liverpool. There were allegations that organs of more than 800 children were removed without the *consent* of their parents during the period between 1988 and 1995.

In the last twenty years, there have been a fairly significant number of cases involving patients' consent to medical interventions. Revising and updating consent forms still goes on in the NHS, some general, but increasingly many being specialty-specific.

References

1. Editorial (Wakefield article linking MMR vaccine and autism was fraudulent), *British Medical Journal*, 2011, **342**, 64-6.
2. Brian Deer, The Lancet's Two Days to Bury Bad News, *British Medical Journal*, 2011, **342**, 200-4.
3. Harvey Marcovitch, Is Research Safe in Their Hands? *British Medical Journal*, 2011, **342**, 206.
4. Luisa Dillner, Regulating Research, *British Medical Journal*, 2011, **342**, 143-4.

5. General Medical Council—Consent and Children, *Guidance for All Doctors* Booklet, October 2007, *www.gmc-uk.org*

6. Dr Karen Roberts, Confidentiality, *MDU Journal*, December 2007, **23**(2), 6-9.

7. Eleaner Peters, M. Challis, Most Doctors See Consent from a Functionalist Perspective, *British Medical Journal*, 1999, **318**, 735.

8. Jeremy Laurence, Medical Research Hit by Sixty Frauds, *The Independent* (UK), 9 September, 1999.

9. Linda Beecham, GMC Advice to Doctors on Consent, *British Medical Journal*, 1999, **318**, 553.

10. Caroline Jones, Communication the Key to Patient Consent, *British Medical Association News Review*, 1999, 15.

11. Deborah Josefson, Informed Consent and Research, *British Medical Journal*, 1998, **316**, 1849.

12. Priscilla Alderson, C. Goody, Theories in Health Care and Research Theories of Consent, *British Medical Journal*, 1998, **317**, 1313-15.

13. Heather Goodare, Studies That Do Not Have Informed Consent from Participants Should Not Be Published, *British Medical Journal*, 1998, **316**, 1004-5.

14. Mary Warnock, Informed Consent—A Publisher's Duty, *British Medical Journal*, 1998, **316**, 1002-3.

15. Richard Smith, Informed Consent, *British Medical Journal*, 1998, **316**, 949-51.

16. Editorial (Informed Consent), *British Medical Association News Review*, January 1998.

17. Saul Radovsky, Bearing the news, *The New England Journal of Medicine*, 1985, **313**(9), 586-8.

Chapter 8

Learning Medical Fallibility

Fallibility is the quality of being fallible, *i.e., liable to err*. Acceptance of and adaptation to one's fallibility is a major part of growth and continued professional competence. However, fear of disclosure of one's mistakes to peers, friends, referring doctors, and patients often prevents doctors from facing the reality of their fallibility. Doctors' recognition of this problem positively affects the daily performance of their duties and may consequently help prevent harm to their patients. If doctors fail to recognise this problem, a pattern of performance detrimental to patients may be reinforced and persist until disaster strikes. Learning to handle medical fallibility can be as important as the mastery of scientific medical knowledge. Fallibility is not limited to age groups, specialty, or range of experience. Dubovsky and Schrier, in 'The Mystique of Medical Training'

(*Journal of the American Medical Association*, 1983, **250**, 3057-8), were correct in stating that the age or experience of the physician is no guarantee that mistakes will be avoided or that anxieties about mistakes will not continue. A doctor's adaptability to his/her fallibility should be encouraged throughout his/her career.

Manifestation of Fallibility

There are many areas in the medical profession where fallibility may manifest itself. One most obvious area is *diagnosis*. Perfection in diagnosis is unattainable with some misdiagnoses being more catastrophic than others. The extent and numbers of misdiagnoses may vary from one specialty to another. Factual ignorance is another area where fallibility creeps in. This includes knowledge about diseases, physical findings, medications, and treatment procedures. Broadly speaking, the state and specialty examination and monitoring boards know and set standard levels of knowledge doctors should have in order to practice efficiently in their chosen medical fields.

Judgement in diagnosis and treatment is yet another area where doctors exhibit fallibility. Decisions such as whether and when to operate, whether a certain type of therapy is to be given, and the timing of all necessary interventions, diagnostic or therapeutic, all of them are potentially bound up in fallibility.

Fox, in *Training for Uncertainty—The Student-Physician* (Harvard University Press, 1957, 204-47), describes in some great detail the uncertainty of all medical knowledge and therapeutics. Technical mishaps also do involve fallibility. Minor omissions or commissions do occur in what may be routine procedures such as inserting central lines, bone marrow aspiration, and other similar invasive interventions. *Illegible handwriting* calls for improvement with dates and times being included and signed. Inappropriate orders or overlooking seemingly minor routines do lead to sometimes devastating effects. Although no doctor can achieve constant success, the failure to always achieve success plagues even the most conscientious of doctors.

For the professional, when in doubt, stop and ask, or abandon whatever you are doing or about to do, if possible.

Common Adaptations to Fallibility

There are several adaptations to fallibility. Some are constructive, but others are unfortunately destructive. In coping with their imperfections, doctors may adopt one or more of several *attitudes* as discussed next.

Callous disregard: This is the most dishonourable and publicly damaging attitude found in the medical profession. It is an attempt by the doctor to cover up his/her mistakes. *Denial* is often concomitant of this attitude. Once set up in this frame of mind, doctors are unlikely to improve, even recognise the need for improvement.

Cynical approach, which is another adaptation to fallibility, involves misrepresentation of concern for the patient. The cynicism is largely an attempt by the doctor to cope with very serious patient complications and the doctor's imperfections. Superficially, this attitude may seem beneficial and appropriate at times, but if not coupled with concern and appropriate resignation about the outcome of all things in life, this attitude is negative and counterproductive.

Bravado or the macho complex may be exhibited by some doctors. Such doctors tend to gloss over their imperfections and mistakes by pointing or stressing the heroic and monumental accomplishments they are trying to achieve.

Excessive guilt is often transitory but incapacitating to doctors for its duration. Doctors may feel unworthy of their professional status. In the overly sensitive, a pattern of excessive concern may develop. Excessive self-scrutiny may paralyse such doctors in their professional duties. Abuse of laboratory, radiological, and other investigative facilities may follow. Indecisions may follow and prolong patients' suffering. Doctors may go on to abandon practice of procedures, thereby denying patients reasonable treatments.

Projection is perhaps the least worthy adaptation to fallibility. It occurs in the obsessive, highly strung doctors who, instead of recognising their own imperfections and failures, do attribute them to other doctors, nurses, and other personnel, worse still to the patient. This behaviour contributes to ill will in those who work with the doctors concerned.

Overwork is yet another attitude a doctor may adopt in an effort to relieve guilt. McCue, in 'The Effects of Stress on Doctors and Their Medical Practice' (New England Journal of Medicine, 1982, **306**, 458-63) describes this attitude by which a doctor may redouble his/her efforts by being on call more often and throwing himself/herself into work in an attempt to show that his/her dedication more than makes up for any imperfections or mistakes. Mistakes then become *misfortunes*. This attitude may lead to a chronic state of dissatisfaction, the end result of which may be an impaired doctor.

Useful guidelines in the recognition and adaptation to one's imperfections may be:

a) By being honest to oneself and to others. This is paramount and has both ethical and legal ramifications. Rather than appear perfect, a mature doctor should freely admit his/her mistakes.

b) Using mistakes as educational tools. Continuing education through books, journals, the Internet, seminars, and through consultations and discussions with senior health-care staff (peers) about complications may help prevent the recurrence of mistakes and limit the behaviour that fosters too many unnecessary mistakes. One can learn more from one's mistakes than his/her successes. In an atmosphere of open discussion, this will actually improve the doctor's patient care.

c) Having compassion is the ultimate in dealing with patient care when mistakes have occurred. This applies to the patient as well as the doctor and his/her peers.

Any adaptation to one's imperfections must deal with the following considerations in medical practice.

Everyone dies. The doctor cannot save everyone or improve or cure everyone's medical problems. No matter how conscientious, well-trained, dedicated, or intelligent a doctor is, he/she is bound to make mistakes, a number of them serious. Not all mistakes are either malpractice or a 'sin'. All teaching programmes should promote honesty and have a personal touch about them. Every conference should include admission to making errors and an honest discussion of mistakes and complications. Personal interviews, as part of training programmes, may expose a doctor's attitude towards fallibility and help cultivate, question, and improve on it. Each mistake or complication should be thoroughly investigated, and as an educational tool, this is indispensable. This should be a continuous practice in the doctor's career.

References

1. Michael Foxton, Medicine Is Driving Us to an Early Grave (Work Stress), *Hospital Doctor*, 17 January, 2002, 18-9.
2. Clare Hughs, Doctors' Handwriting: The Write Stuff, *Hospital Doctor*, 17 October, 2002, *http://www.global* 2000.net/handwriting repair

3. Daniel H. Carmichael, Learning Medical Fallibility, *Southern Medical Journal*, 1985, **78**(1), 1-3.

4. David Hilfiker, Facing Our Mistakes, *The New England Journal of Medicine*, 1984, **310**, 118-22.

5. Dubovsky and Schrier, The Mystique of Medical Training, *Journal of the American Medical Association*, 1983, **250**, 3057-8.

6. Fox, *Training for Uncertainty—The Student-Physician*, Harvard University Press, 1957, 204-47.

Chapter 9

Psychology of Medical Disasters:
Risk Assessment of Medical Disasters

Disasters bring human terror, anguish, and despair—anguish at the occurrence of the disaster and despair when one realises life can never be the same again. Psychological debriefing after a disaster is vital. Powell, in 1954, described a model of psychological manifestations based on the following phases:

Warning phase, during which one may recognise that conditions are present which could lead to disaster, e.g., a wrong diagnosis, wrong treatment or non-treatment.

Threat phase is when there are specific indicators of an impending disaster. This is the phase when one realises that something wrong is happening, e.g., when the wrong operation is taking place or more than planned and consented surgery is occurring.

Impact phase is when it all happens. The patient has received the wrong drug(s), wrong dosage, or the patient has had the wrong operation or dangerous anaesthetic. When the patient has come to harm or is dead, the following phases of psychological reactions come into play, namely, *Inventory, Rescue, Remedy,* and *Recovery.*

Inventory phase is when the doctor concerned takes stock of what has happened to him/her and to the patient. There is exhibition of shock, fear, and panic.

Rescue phase is when colleagues come to console the doctor concerned and help him/her to a shelter, preferably his/her home.

Remedy phase is when specific formal steps are taken to help the doctor deal with the aftermath of the disaster.

Recovery phase is the very long subsequent period in which the doctor adjusts to his/her altered personal circumstances. It includes coming to terms with the experience of the disaster.

This model provides the framework for thinking about behaviour, emotional experiences, and psychological suffering of people caught up in personal or general disaster situations. Few of us spend time thinking about the disaster which may happen to us. We live and work in a potentially dangerous environment, but if we were to constantly be fearful and watch for something dreadful to happen, we would do little else. Many individuals not only do not think about the possibility of a disaster but will act, even under conditions of great risk, as though the disaster could not possibly happen to them. Many of these individuals appear to carry with them a sense of personal invulnerability.

Risk assessment and Medical Disasters

When we do contemplate the possibility of an accident or disaster, we weigh up the nature of the threat and the various risks. This involves asking questions like these:

How many times has it happened before? If nothing of the sort has happened before, there is little likelihood of a proper risk assessment taking place.

What would happen to me? The answer to this question may ring alarm bells but may not trigger a risk assessment exercise. Facing the victim's relatives would send a shudder down every doctor's spine.

What are the most likely effects to my family and others? Shame seems to be an immediate deterrent, but loss of a job and livelihood is a more formidable aftermath which would affect the family directly and be noticed and discussed by others. A trip to the General Medical Council (UK) and to the courts would certainly mark a grave situation.

What are the possible effects to staff at the workplace and residence, and how severe might these effects be? In the beginning, there is solidarity. All will rally round the doctor in this time of need. The immediate family members and close friends would offer help of all sorts. Some will follow developments for a while and then abandon the doctor.

Survival behaviour: There is pro-social behaviour which leads to helping or sharing in order to survive. Longing for loved ones contributes to the 'will to live'. Praying, even for those who have never believed in a benign deity, will be by one begging a power outside oneself to save one. Also to occur may be bargaining with *God* or *Fate,* saying, 'Just get me out of this and I will . . .' Response of hope is defined as 'active longing for rescue'. *Hope* functions to control mood by promoting the belief that what is happening cannot last.

Psychological factors in the Rescue and Remedy phases: During these two phases, stress is acute in the doctor and other medical personnel of a team. In a medical incident, the stressors are acute or subacute, but the response to them may have a very long time span. Selye, in 1956, saw stress as a 'non-specific physiological response' in which an individual reacts to a stressor, first with alarm and then with resistance. If the stressor continues, resistance eventually deteriorates and bodily resources are used up. In extreme cases, collapse and death may ensue. Selye believed that the stress response did not depend on the nature of the stressor and represented a universal pattern of defence reactions serving to protect an individual and preserve his/her integrity. This is called the General Adaptation Syndrome (GAS). Stress which exceeds the limit of the inbuilt resistance results in permanent physiological and psychological damage.

Psychological factors in the Recovery phase: These factors are related to serious injury to or loss of a patient. The loss of a *job* and *income,* loss of *social status,* and loss of *friends* are dominant thoughts during this period.

These thoughts often lead an individual to fall ill and he/she may even become physically ill. A previously well-balanced and resourceful doctor may be driven into a state of 'madness' in which he/she fears for his/her sanity.

Post-traumatic Stress Disorder

An individual involved in a disaster may become unable to fulfil everyday roles which may have to be taken over by other members of the team. A 'safe holding environment', which allows the doctor to talk freely about his/her experiences without risk of being blamed, judged, criticised, or have others impose their interpretations or definitions about what the doctor has experienced, should be provided. Psychological support has to be aimed at encouraging this process of working through experiences by talking about them, recognising the emotions experienced, and accepting them.

Psychological Aftercare

The process of adjusting after a disaster is a long one and the need for reality-testing by talking about the 'incident' to sympathetic people is very real. Such people need to have a professional understanding of and experience in what has happened and the emotions involved. The doctor's relatives and friends may grow tired of hearing repeated accounts of his/her experience and may prematurely tell him/her to stop raking it over.

'Pull yourself together' may be the advice, and the cry 'it still hurts' may fall on deaf ears.

References

1. T. Cox and C. J. McKay, A Psychological Model of Occupational Stress, *Medical Research Council Meeting*, London, 1976.
2. B. Raphael, *When Disaster Strikes: A Handbook for the Caring profession*, C. Hutchinson, London.

3. H. Kay, Accidents: Some Facts and Theories, *Psychology at Work*, Penguin Books, 1971.
4. I. L. Javis, et al., Emergency Decision-making—A Theoretical Analysis of Responses to Disaster Warnings, *Journal of Human Stress*, 1977, **3**, 35-45.

Chapter 10

Doctors' professional obligations to their Patients

Doctors claim to have special supererogatory moral obligations to their patients, that is, moral obligations that are over and above the ordinary moral obligations we all have to each other. Some prima facie moral duties of doctors to their patients and their implications are briefly discussed here, excluding the manifold problems that arise when these obligations conflict.

First is the principle of autonomy: In their relationship with patients, doctors must remember that apart from any special moral obligations, they have the standard moral obligations that all of us have to each other—to respect each other's autonomy, not to harm each other (*non-malfeasance*), to be just, and to benefit others (*beneficence*). In addition, doctors voluntarily take on additional moral obligations which might be called 'principle of medical beneficence'. This is to benefit their patients' health and, to some extent, the health of others. Doctors undertake to do so by trying to save their patients' lives when these lives are threatened by disease and other maladies, to cure, palliate, prevent maladies, and to ameliorate the suffering that these cause.

Doctors' general duty to respect their patients' autonomy requires that if the patient does not want to be helped, doctors generally have no right to help them (with certain exceptions). Even the general doctors' duty not to harm others requires, for the most part, that they try their best to obtain their patients' willing and informed consent to what is proposed as most interventions designed to help others carry a risk of harming, and this risk is increased considerably if interventions are carried out without the patients' understanding and consent, let alone if these interventions are carried out against their will.

Doctors may advise but their patients should be given the opportunity to decide whether or not to accept their advice. A patient's rejection of medical advice should not lead to a shrugging of the shoulders. What should follow instead is a genuine attempt to understand the patient's reason for rejecting the advice. The special obligation of medical *beneficence* reinforces the doctor's duty to respect their patients' autonomy. Doctors would benefit their patients more if the rationale of their proposed beneficial actions is understood and approved by their patients.

One of the key factors to respecting patients' autonomy is *good communication*. Thus, doctors need to acquire and maintain skills in communicating with their patients. Other prima facie obligations deriving from the principle of respect for autonomy may include the provision of more information about doctors' interests, qualifications, attitudes, and moral stances to patients as well as making it easy for patients to have a real choice of doctors. In practice, this is still a very difficult goal to achieve. Here in the UK, it has been difficult for 'problem patients' who wish to change doctors to do so. Respect for autonomy of the patient would seem at first sight to require otherwise. The General Medical Council advised against specialists accepting patients without referral by their general practitioners (GPs). The same general council, however, went on to state that ' . . . an individual patient is *free* to seek to consult any doctor'. The World Medical Association, in the Declaration of Lisbon, goes on to say, 'The patient has the right to choose his/her doctor freely.'

Shared decisions in which patients and health professionals join, in both the process of decision-making and ownership of the decisions made, has attracted considerable interest as a means by which patients' preferences can be incorporated into clinical decisions. When there are several treatment options which may have different effects on the patients' quality of life, there is a strong case for offering patients choice, and it must be informed choice. Patients cannot express informed preferences unless they are given sufficient and appropriate information including detailed explanations about their conditions and the likely outcomes with or without treatment.

Many patients still report some difficulties in obtaining relevant medical information. There is a number of reasons for this happening. Health professionals frequently underestimate the patients' desire for and ability to cope with medical information when presented in a non-alarmist fashion, is balanced, and includes a careful and honest assessment of pros and cons of treatment. Consultation times are short and limited, and therefore, there is insufficient time to explain fully the condition and treatment choices.

A solution to this problem is to ensure that patients have access to and do understand written or audiovisual patients' materials. These materials should not contain inaccuracies or misleading statements which could give false impressions of the likely effectiveness of treatments. The most common fault is to give an over-optimistic view, emphasising only benefits and glossing over risks and side effects. Qualitative information about recovery times and outcome probabilities may be absent from some of these materials. Information in these materials may not admit to scientific uncertainty or variations in clinical opinion. It is important that patient information is based on the best and most up to date medical knowledge available about treatment and research. Materials which give patients a sense of empowerment are most likely to be popular. These may include materials which reassure patients that they are not alone in experiencing the symptoms—materials which give patients ideas for self-help and materials which have suggestions as to which questions to ask their doctors during consultations.

Patients' materials should have answers to the following questions and worries:

What is causing the problem and am I alone?
How does my experience compare with that of other patients?
Is there anything I can do to ameliorate the problem?
What is the purpose of tests and investigations?
What are the different treatment options?
What are the benefits of the treatments?
What are the risks of the treatments?
Is it essential to have treatment for this condition?
Will the treatment relieve the symptoms?
How long will it take to recover?
What are the possible side effects, and what effect will the treatment have on sex life?
How can one prepare for the treatment?
What are the procedures followed when one goes into hospital?

When can one leave hospital?
What do carers need to know?
What can one do to speed up recovery?
What are the options for rehabilitation?
How can one prevent recurrence or future illness?
Where can one get more information about the problem or treatment?

Second and Third principles are: non-malfeasance (not to harm each other*)* and *beneficence* (benefiting others). These two principles refer to the doctor-patient relationship, and they are considered together, for although non-malfeasance can be considered independently of beneficence, any obligation to help others that may result in harm, including almost any medical intervention, has to be considered in the context of the coexisting obligation 'not to harm others'. Countless important prima facie medical obligations stem from these two principles, of which the following are a few:

a) If the doctor professes to be able and willing to benefit his/her patients, then he/she had better be able and willing to do so.
b) As the doctor is under obligation not to harm others, he/she had better carry out his/her duties with minimal harm to his/her patients.

By accepting these two principles, doctors are obliged to ensure that they practice in ways that do actually benefit their patients with minimal harm. Thus, improving clinical practice standards, with continuing medical education and professional development, with some form of audit, is a moral obligation as distinct from an extra one taken on by the enthusiasts.

Closing ranks in individual and group interests against the interests of patients is incompatible with the adherence to a principle of benefiting patients (beneficence).

When a doctor makes a mistake, he/she has a duty to *say sorry* to the patient. This requirement may in any case be of considerable benefit to the doctor as well as to the victim of his/her mistake. All doctors are nice to some of their patients some of the time, and patients would prefer a medically competent but unpleasant doctor to a charming ignoramus. These are not mutually exclusive. Beneficence requires only good feelings, and doctors should exhibit 'moderate love' for their patients.

References

1. Tony Delamothe, When Things Go Wrong, *British Medical Journal*, 2009, **339**, b4226.
2. Daniel. K. Sokol, Can Deceiving Patients Be Morally Acceptable? *British Medical Journal*, 2007, **334**, 984-6.
3. General Medical Council, Charter of Understanding between Doctors and People Affected by Medical Accidents, *General Medical Council News*, 19 August, 2003, 8, *www.gmc-uk.org*
4. Dr Sally Barnard, Love and the Hospital Doctor, *Hospital Doctor*, 24 October, 2002, 42, *www.hospital-doctor.net*
5. Angela Coulter, V. Entwistle, and D. Gilbert, Sharing Decisions with Patients: Is the Information Good Enough? *British Medical Journal*, 1999, **318**, 318-22.
6. Raanan Gillon, Physicians and Patients, *British Medical Journal*, 1986, **292**, 466-9.

Chapter 11

Doctor-Patient relationship:
Its effect on the Outcome of
Medical Errors and Adverse Events

Little has been written concerning the impact of an iatrogenic complication or adverse outcome on the doctor-patient relationship. Underlying good doctor-patient relationship is the foundation on which medical error or adverse event occurs. The adverse event is a critical stressor that can either undermine or ultimately strengthen the relationship. Both the previous nature of the relationship and the actual management of the adverse event when it occurs will influence the ultimate course of events.

Three components of the doctor-patient relationship seem to determine the type of reaction to an adverse event a patient may exhibit.

a) The style of interaction and communication between the patient and the doctor.

The doctor-patient interaction can vary as follows: The interaction can be a passive-active relationship, where the doctor determines what is to be done or said and the patient passively accepts it. The interaction may be a guidance-cooperation one, where the doctor basically tells the patient what should be done and the patient usually concurs. Finally, the interaction may be of a mutual partnership to make decisions and work on problems together. There is a sharing of information and risks. The more dominant the doctor's role, the greater the likelihood that the patient could blame the doctor should an adverse event occur.

b) The handling of uncertainty in decision-making and informed consent.

Informed consent means more than a signature on a form. As previously discussed under 'informed consent', patients must be given sufficient information to understand the procedures to be carried out and be fully aware of what can go wrong. If these requirements have not been met and something goes wrong, the patient is inclined to *complain* or *sue* and the door is open for litigation lawyers. Doctors are not legally obliged to tell their patients all details of their treatment but only that information that a 'responsible body of doctors' would believe is appropriate to give. The General Medical Council (UK) was of the view that, irrespective of the legality of the circumstances, there is an ethical requirement for a doctor to be open and frank to his/her patients. One, however, should always keep in mind the anxiety some types of information may cause the patient.

c) The degree to which a trust relationship has been established between the patient and doctor.

Good communication between patient and doctor is important for patient satisfction, and therefore, the patient's reaction to the adverse event may depend on the *degree* of communication. Patients' expectations and concerns need receive great attention if dissatisfaction is to be minimised. The patient's attitude towards the doctor's conduct is especially influenced by the doctor's offer of information important to the patient; the thoroughness of information-gathering; the doctor concerned taking preventive measures to avoid or minimise risks; and last but not least, the doctor being prudent.

Patients turn to doctors both to get treated for their illnesses and also to get help to change their uncertainty and fears to *certainty* and *hope*. Once an adverse event has occurred, both the patient and the doctor must sort through issues and resolve any potential problems that can be a threat to the continued good doctor-patient relationship.

Problems related to the Patient in Doctor-Patient relationship

The patient may feel that the doctor is the cause of, or at least, the agent for his/her suffering. The patient may subconsciously blame the doctor even if the patient consciously admits the decision that led to the adverse event was warranted at the time. Chronic suffering or incapacity may generate a deep sense of anger or hostility. This anger may be focused on the doctor concerned or be projected to his/her colleagues and thereby affect future professional relationships. When trust is impaired, the patient may be inhibited in openly communicating his/her anxieties, fears, or anger to the doctor. If the patient's concerns are not addressed, he/she may cease all efforts to communicate. The patient may blame himself/herself for agreeing with the decision that led to the adverse event. These feelings of fate may lead the patient to accept his/her lot and never express the anguish to the doctor.

If the patient feels the doctor is not appropriately concerned and communication is inadequate or the doctor feels the patient is not adequately committed to the relationship, either party may begin to terminate the relationship. Patients who feel ignored or rejected by their doctors are more likely to *complain* and consider a *lawsuit* as a way of forcing the doctor to share in the responsibility and experience the anger and suffering resulting from the adverse event.

Problems related to the Doctor in Doctor-Patient relationship

Various factors may cause the doctor to provide inappropriate management of a situation following the occurrence of an adverse event. The doctor may see the adverse event as a threat to his/her identity as a *healer* with *power* and *control* over disease and patients. The doctor's feelings of responsibility for the adverse outcome may engender (arouse or stir up) feelings of guilt and professional or personal inadequacy. Doctors who have maintained a doctor-dominant style of interaction with their patients may attempt to restructure the doctor-patient relationship, doctor-patient interactions, and limit effective communication. Finally, the doctor may fear that the patient with an adverse outcome may sue. Such fears may inhibit the doctor from being candid about the exact nature or cause of the adverse event. The doctor may even deny that the adverse event is real. In these circumstances, communication will often be seriously impaired and the risk of malpractice suit may increase.

Patients' Expectations of Doctors to handle the Aftermath of Medical Errors and Adverse Events

A large number of patients desire some acknowledgement of even minor errors. For moderate to severe errors, patients are more likely to consider *litigation* if the doctor does not disclose the error. Patients want full disclosure whatever the severity of the error. Disclosure may reduce the risk of punitive actions by patients in general, and open communication between doctor and patient becomes critical indeed.

There are many ways a doctor may communicate the bad news to his/her patient. They include the following:

a) *Simple expression of sympathy* as appropriate as it does not equate with admission of liability, yet it shows the doctor's true concern for the situation. It is a moral imperative for a doctor to honestly acknowledge his/her mistakes. Only then can a doctor begin to make constructive changes in his/her practice to avoid these mistakes in the future.

b) *Full disclosure* to patients and if appropriate, to their relatives. Most authorities are in agreement that a patient has a right to full disclosure. Anything less could undermine the doctor-patient relationship in the long run. This is the only way the doctor can achieve a sense of absolution.

c) *Corrective action taken*—the medical profession must take a more vigorous and creative role in reducing errors that occur. Mistakes are inevitable in medical practice given its inherent uncertainty and complexity, and the need to make decisions despite limited information. Doctors should learn from their mistakes even as they strive to minimise their occurrence.

Ways to help learn from mistakes and institute constructive changes in practice should include the following:

- Accepting responsibility for one's mistakes even though this inevitably leads to emotional distress for the doctor concerned

- Discussing mistakes with *colleagues*, especially *peers* who are legally and ethically responsible for overall patient care
- Reducing workload to minimise *fatigue* and resultant *stress*
- Keeping up to date by attending relevant courses under continuing medical education and continuing professional development programmes
- Retraining or a change of specialty or career if appropriate

References

1. Garbutt, et al., Reporting and Disclosing Medical Errors: Pediatricians' Attitudes and Behaviours, *Archives of Pediatrics & Adolescent Medicine*, 2007, **161**, 179-85.
2. Dr Anahita Kirkpatrick, Ian Baker, When Patients Love—or Hate—You, *MDU Journal*, April 2003, **19**, 20-1.
3. A. B. Witman, et al., How Do Patients Want Physicians to Handle Mistakes? *Archives of Pediatrics & Adolescent Medicine*, 1996, **156**, 2565-9.
4. Albert W. Wu, et al., Do House Officers Learn from Their Mistakes? *Journal of the American Medical Association*, 1991, **265**(16), 2089-94.
5. William P. Applegate, Physician Management of Patients with Adverse Outcomes, *Archives of Internal Medicine*, 1986, **146**, 2249-52.

Chapter 12

Doctors' response to Medical Error Outcomes: Mechanisms used to cope with the Aftermath

Doctors have major, sometimes sole, responsibility for patient health care. They are constantly cognisant of the heavy demands this responsibility does involve. They are deeply aware of the variety of factors which can contribute to less than satisfactory, and sometimes, catastrophic outcomes for patients under their management. Unanticipated problems do emerge every day, ultimately contributing to tension and fear in many doctors. Serious and fatal errors are made by doctors during some stage of their careers. Painfully, doctors are even less prepared to deal with their mistakes than the average layperson is. The climate of medical school and house officer training, for instance, makes it nearly impossible to confront the emotional consequences of mistakes. The environment in which doctors are trained does not encourage them to talk openly about their mistakes or to talk about emotional responses to their mistakes. The medical profession seems to have no place for its own mistakes. If the profession has no room for its mistakes, society seems to have even more rigid expectations of its doctors. The word 'malpractice' carries with it the implication that one has done something more than make a natural mistake. It connotes guilt and sinfulness.

The potential consequences of medical mistakes are so overwhelming that it is almost impossible for practicing doctors to deal with errors in a psychologically healthy fashion. Most people, doctors and patients alike, harbour deep within themselves the expectation that the doctor will always be perfect. No one seems to accept the simple fact of life that doctors, like anyone else, will err. Doctors are not *paragons* of virtue. By the very nature of their work, doctors daily make decisions of extreme gravity. Their work in places like **Intensive Care Units** (or Intensive Therapy Units), **Accident and Emergency** units, or **Obstetric Units**, and the **Operating Theatres**, to mention but a few, offers doctors lots of opportunities daily to miscalculate, often with disastrous consequences. At some point in their practice, doctors must bring mistakes out of the closet. They need to give themselves permission to recognise their errors and consequences. Doctors need to find healthy ways to deal with their emotional responses to those errors. Their profession is difficult enough without their having to *wear the yoke of perfection.*

Doctors are devastated by serious mistakes that harm or kill their patients. The emotional impact is often profound, typically a mixture of fear, guilt, anger, embarrassment, and humiliation. Doctors are, however, typically isolated by their emotional responses. Seldom is there a proper process to evaluate the circumstances of a mistake and to provide support and emotional healing for the fallible doctor. Guilty feelings may interfere with the doctor's professional performance and personal well-being. Feelings of guilt may result in rumination on the event, self-doubt, and personal anguish. The severity of the outcome of an error plays a key role in the doctor's resultant feelings. Perceptions of other people also influence the doctor's feelings of guilt. If the patient and his/her family think the doctor has made a mistake or openly criticise his/her care, he/she will tend to ruminate more about the episode. These feelings are a result of internal distress about disappointing the patient and the doctor's own inadequacies.

Physicians get worried about the perceptions of colleagues because they do not want their peers to think poorly of their quality of care. They need support and more understanding of their colleagues and patients when they make mistakes.

Doctor's response to the occurrence of medical error may include the following:

The doctor may accept responsibility for the adverse outcome, promising to do things differently next time round and to take advice.

He/she may take to criticising or lecturing to oneself, or to apologising and doing something to make up.

The doctor may discuss the adverse event and its outcome with the patient and /or with the patient's family member(s).

He/she may discuss the occurrence with colleagues, both temporary and peers.

He/she may contact non-medical personnel like the chaplain or counsellor.

He/she may refer the matter to his/her medical defence organisation for advice and help.

Some doctors may decide to discuss the case at a medical conference or at such relevant professional meetings.

Finally, a doctor may decide against telling anyone about the event.

The realities of the malpractice threat provide strong incentive against disclosure or the proper handling and investigation of mistakes. Even a minor error could place the doctor's entire career in jeopardy if it later results in a serious outcome.

Mechanisms Doctors may use to cope with the Aftermath of Medical Errors

The following is a framework for managing stressful circumstances and possible deviant behaviour which may accompany the occurrence of medical errors and adverse events.

The coping mechanism is defined as 'healthy adaptations under stress'. The doctor deals efficiently and professionally in solving the outcomes of an error or adverse event.

The defence mechanism is defined as 'adaptive devices gone wrong' so that the cognitive field is either partially blocked out or subjected to a major interpretive distortion. However, *sociological* definitions of defence mechanisms as opposed to *psychological* mechanisms include a greater interaction and learned element—more situational and less as an innate, idiosyncratic, and permanent part of self. Vacillating between healthy and unhealthy processes may be exhibited by the doctor to his/her mistakes.

The defences against problems which arise during patient management are as follows:

The denial process is a neutralisation technique also known as 'denial of injury'. It is a defence mechanism which is entrenched in the medical profession. It is both employed as a disclaimer and as an account providing a behavioural repertoire for handling past and future events. Denial is manifested by the following modes of behaviour.

a) Negation of the concept of error by identifying the practice of medicine as a 'grey area'. Denial is part of the 'clinical orientation or clinical mentality' in the practice of medicine. It includes individualisation of cases, since each one is different. It also includes the belief that 'medicine is as much an art as is a science'. Many of the mistakes committed may therefore be redefined as non-mistakes.

b) Repression (i.e., forgetting what occurred) is another type of denial which involves blocking out the mistake from one's consciousness.

c) Redefinition of a mistake as non-mistake is common among doctors. They narrow the definition of mistakes by excluding many so-called 'minor ones'. This allows doctors to admit only to some of the errors while dismissing others as inconsequential.

The discounting process: When the errors cannot be denied because of the magnitude of the outcome, the doctor may utilise a variety of elaborate mechanisms by which he/she discounts his/her responsibility and thereby exonerates himself/herself to varying degrees. This is called 'denial of responsibility'. In this way, the doctor defends himself/herself by externalising the blame, at least in part, to someone else or something other than himself/herself. This may include blaming the bureaucratic system outside of medicine, his/her superiors or subordinates or other colleagues within medicine, the disease, and finally, the patient.

By blaming the system, the rationale is that, although doctors knew what should or could have been done to prevent the error, they blame lack of time, tiredness, or hassle for their failure to stop it happening. Given the amount of work a doctor has to do and the obstacles to be confronted, he/she often feels justified in performing under par.

Blaming the superiors: A junior doctor may pass the responsibility for the error up the chain of command. He/she may attempt to partially exonerate himself/herself by pointing to the fact that more experienced doctors in the system are not faultless. However, junior doctors blaming their superiors or supervisors as a discounting mechanism, raises questions about responsibility and authority which have serious consequences both for patient care and staff relationships. Occasionally, junior doctors will be blamed for the errors committed by their seniors, usually when advice was not sought from the seniors before undertaking difficult tasks.

Blaming the disease, the patient and the science of medicine: A doctor resigns himself/herself to the fact that certain disease processes are irreversible and untreatable. There are limitations in medicine. This attitude makes the doctor discount his/her sense of culpability. A doctor may view his/her error within the context of personal lack of medical knowledge and the lack of collective knowledge in his/her field of medicine. This type of blame also consists of a demonstration to the effect that no one else knew how to handle this particular situation. Therefore, the doctor was personally ignorant. 'He should not have known better' because no one else did either. The doctor may blame the patient for not revealing sufficient information about the current or past medical history and problems in it so that the doctor could make a correct diagnosis and give the corrective treatment. Then, the patient's honesty and discipline comes into question. Finally a patient may be the one 'blamed' for not getting better in spite of the best treatment provided or for doing worse and deteriorating. The overweight, the smoker, the alcoholic, and the drug addict patient may fall into this category.

Distancing mechanisms: These are employed when the doctor can no longer deny or discount an error because of its magnitude. Profound doubts and even guilt—feelings which do not easily or automatically resolve themselves remain to haunt the doctor. Fundamental questions of culpability and responsibility intersperse among the doctor's defences as he/she vacillates between self and others to blame. A doctor may come to a point when he/she can neither deny nor discount errors made. Hence, he/she acquires a third set of responses to protect himself/herself from the repercussions of serious mistakes and to lessen his/her sense of guilt and responsibility. This process known as 'distancing' includes a variety of shared beliefs allowing a direct admission of guilt. Justifications include the contention that 'everyone makes mistakes'; 'it could not be helped'; 'I did the best I could.' After all, regardless of the acquisition of knowledge, skills, and values, there still remains the elusive issue of chance.

Temporary versus Permanent resolution of Medical Errors

Coping and *defence* mechanisms, (i.e. *denial, discounting, and distancing*), are acquired and shared self-perceptions about errors of patient management which evolve during advanced medical training. The whole process of managing medical errors, including defining and defending them, is an ambiguous process. Utilising these mechanisms does not necessarily exonerate a doctor from self or other blame. Use of the various mechanisms seems to depend more on the type of error than on the level of seniority of the doctor concerned. The more serious the error, the more heavily the full force of the repertoire is invoked. Utilisation of these techniques does not fully shield a doctor from the guilt or shame felt or keep doubts and ambivalence from surfacing, even if the doctor is not always fully cognisant of their adverse effects. While a doctor may feel guilty and remorseful over the error made, he/she would have developed elaborate mechanisms of distancing and denial which, while not completely successful psychologically, are artefacts of a highly insular and self-protective subculture. A doctor who successfully copes with error and its aftermath may tend to be insensitive to the intra-psychic experience and orient himself/herself more to his/her inner world.

Accountability of Doctors

Bergman, in 1981, defined *accountability* from a set of preconditions, mainly three:

The first precondition is 'ability', which refers to *knowledge* of, *skills* of, and *values* of the participant.

The second precondition is 'responsibility', which refers to *tasks* and *roles* undertaken and *duties* assigned to the participant.

The third precondition is 'authority', which refers to the freedom and degree of making and acting on decisions in the exercise of one's professional role.

Accountability refers to a position in which a health-care professional has direct responsibility and is answerable for his/her actions. It may also be defined as a process by which such professionals are judged within legal and ethical boundaries.

Modes of Accountability

There are four distinct modes of accountability in health-care practice. They are *self, legal, contractual,* and *professional* modes.

Self mode of accountability is the moral dimension which cannot be enforced legally. It is the instinctive sense of right or wrong possessed by people. If one possesses knowledge, skills, and experience, one should be capable of differentiating right from wrong. Marks Maran, in 1993, argued that the self mode of accountability is the identification and clarification of one's personal values—what is right or wrong for one.

Legal mode of accountability is one of the external modes of accountability. The law surrounds all aspects of life in every society, and health care is no exception. Legal mode of accountability can be divided into *criminal law* and *civil law.* Health-care professionals are accountable to the public through the criminal law and to the patient through the civil law here in the UK. However, there have been cases where health-care professionals have been convicted of civil offences committed while they were undertaking their professional duties.

Contractual mode of accountability involves the relationship between the doctor and his/her employer. This is sometimes called 'formal accountability'. It is the allegiance of the doctor to his/her employer and to his/her patients. It means that legally, the doctor has to carry out the 'reasonable' orders of the employer if they fall within the guidance of the policies, procedures, and standards the employer set.

Professional mode of accountability is to do with patient safety protection. This mode of accountability is overseen by a professional body, the principle function of which is to maintain a medical register of qualified and competent professionals and to remove those who are unfit to practice. A code of conduct provides the guiding principles by which professionals are held accountable and judged by. This is known as 'professional law'. Being accountable to a professional body is the toughest external mode of accountability, certainly tougher than legal and contractual obligations.

Different modes of accountability can be seen to converge within given practice situations, but these modes essentially work in different ways. A key difference between legal and professional modes of accountability is that the law of negligence is concerned with setting the *minimum standard* of care, whereas professional law is concerned with promoting the *highest standards* of health care. The professional mode of accountability is the toughest on the individual doctor, and therefore it is superior to legal and contractual modes.

Informal mode of accountability is that to colleagues, both subordinates and peers. Doctors believe that only colleagues are the appropriate group of people to assess their errors, if only with great caution and within narrowly defined parameters. Sanctions by any other person, when doctors err, may be unwelcome and judged inappropriate. A doctor may see himself/herself as the sole arbiter of mistakes and their adjudication. He/she may develop a *strong ideology* justifying his/her jealously guarded autonomy. Because of the doctor's privileged position, his/her aura of technical expertise, and the reticence of others within the larger system to judge him/her, this strong ideology is reinforced by a social structure which is ambiguous concerning doctors' accountability for their actions. Doctors are being held accountable for their mistakes by outside agencies, usually following the occurrence of gross errors which could not be overlooked, when patients or their families sue, and when criminal negligence or intent is uncovered.

References

1. Leonard, Patient Safety and Quality Improvement: Medical Errors and Adverse Events, *Pediatric Review*, **31**, 2010, 151-8.
2. Dr Jannet Page, How My Life and Career Were Affected by One Error, *Hospital Doctor*, November 2001, 26-9.
3. Dr Raj Persaud, How to Cope with the Stress of a Patient's Death, *Hospital Doctor*, August 2000, 30-31, *www.hospital-doctor.net*
4. Dr Raj Persaud : How to cope with patient's death, British Medical Journal 320, 2000:1571-4.

5. Prof. Lucian Leape, Error in Medicine, *Journal of the American Medical Association*, **272**(23), 1994, 1851-7.

6. Albert W. Wu, S. Folkman et al. Do House Officers Learn from their Mistakes? *Journal of the American Medical Association*, **265**(16), 1991, 2089-94.

7. Wendy Levison, Patrick M. Dunn, et al., Copying with Fallibility, *Journal of the American Medical Association*, **261**(15), 1989, 2252.

8. David Hilfiker, Facing Our Mistakes, *The New Engl. J. Med.* **310**, 1984, 118-22.

Chapter 13

Managing the Aftermath of Medical Errors and Adverse Events: Cleaning up afterwards and reducing the threat of Litigation

The basic components for the proper management of medical errors and adverse clinical outcomes are as follows.

Informed Consent, Sufficient patient participation in decision-making, patient's knowledge of risks and uncertainty involved in his/her clinical management.

With these three components satisfied, the patient's reaction to the adverse outcome is likely to be less damaging to the doctor-patient relationship. Regardless of previous events, once an adverse event has occurred, full disclosure of its nature is necessary. Lack of disclosure will usually undermine the doctor-patient relationship over time and greatly influence his/her decision to seek legal redress. As previously discussed, the patient has the right to full disclosure of his/her medical problems unless that patient is incompetent, or disclosure would cause the patient immediate harm. In the majority of cases, it is unlikely that disclosure of the truth would be as disabling as suffering from adverse symptoms in a state of uncertainty.

The doctor should not minimise or deny the problem as this will result in the patient feeling that his/her relationship with the doctor is impaired or limited. Ongoing open communication with the patient and encouragement to express his/her concerns, fears, and anger must be maintained. This way the doctor will be in a strong position to correct any misconceptions the patient may harbour without losing credibility or trust. Uncertainty about the course of future events should be acknowledged and emphasised with the patient. The doctor should give as optimistic and as realistic an appraisal of events as possible under the prevailing circumstances. Adequate time must be allowed for patient's visits to allow frank interchange to take place. This way the patient may feel his/her needs are being met despite the adverse outcome. Sometimes frank and open communication with the patient over an adverse outcome may strengthen the relationship over time, once the initial emotional reaction to the event is worked through.

The doctor must, from time to time, assess his/her feelings about the adverse event and its outcomes and analyse any influence such feelings may have on his/her behaviour towards the patient. Follow-up appointments must be made and patient's contacts strengthened with prompt action. When deemed necessary, consultations with other doctors or medical teams should be sought. If a consultation is with another doctor, the referring doctor should describe clearly the reasons for the consultation and express a wish for the patient to return to his/her care afterwards. This way the patient may be inclined to try to work through his/her clinical problems with the doctor concerned.

Sometimes, however, despite these efforts, it will not be possible to maintain adequate doctor-patient relationship. Lingering resentments on the part of the patient may hamper and eventually permanently damage the relationship. Open discussion may reveal to the doctor that his/her patient has irrevocably lost confidence in him/her. Even at this stage, painful to the doctor as it may be, the matter must be managed with the patient's interest at heart.

The doctor, after carefully examining his/her motives prior to making this recommendation, should advise the patient that other medical practitioners ready to take over her care are available. The final decision on whether or not to terminate the relationship should be left to the patient so that he/she does not feel he/she has been driven away. The doctor should provide the patient with names and addresses of other doctors and allow sufficient time for the patient to make the necessary decision and arrangements. The doctor should take the liberty to express his/her wish to see the patient at any time in the future, if and when appropriate.

Cleaning up after Medical Errors and Adverse Events

As medical errors and adverse events occurring during medical treatment continue to occur, an increasing number of patients desire some acknowledgement of even minor errors. Failure by the doctor to disclose the error to the patient may exhibit a variety of reactions as discussed under doctor-patient rapport. Acknowledgement of the error may lead to the patient accepting it with an *apology* and continue with the relationship with the doctor, or the patient may request a referral to another doctor. The severe the error or adverse the event outcome, the more the desire for the patient to report and file a lawsuit with or without demand for financial compensation. The patient may go to court in spite of receiving 'proper' management from the doctor concerned or from any other relevant medical personnel.

The key to minimising problems after a medical mishap is *good communication*. When the worst happens, the patient has been harmed by the doctor; the discussion which follows will throw some light on how to handle the aftermath. By good communication the majority of legal actions could be avoided or minimised. The doctor should keep control of the situation and thereby reduce the great stress caused by the tragedy. A number of useful steps should be taken to help prevent needless litigation, improve doctor-patient and doctor-relatives relationships, and preserve the doctor's mental health and protect him/her if and when litigation does take place.

A major adverse event produces a lot of emotions, and the legal implications are far from certain. In these circumstances, the need for open communication extends to the next of kin, hospital staff, referring doctors, the legal personnel, as well as the doctor's family. Where informed consent is obtained by the doctor and the patient and his/her family are warned of potential problems, the aftermath can and should be controllable because most of those involved will have been prepared for the poor outcome or for the occurrence of the adverse events. It is not suggested that informed consent protects a doctor from the consequences of medical error or adverse event, but with informed consent, the patient's and his/her family's expectations and acceptance of what has happened will be based on what was in the informed consent. Where informed consent was not obtained by the doctor, the aftermath will be already out of control. A number of emotions ranging from guilt, fear, anger, numbness, and a sense of loss would hit the doctor and his/her team members following an adverse event. The patient's next of kin would have assumed or been informed that the procedure or treatment is safe or without significant risk.

Gravity of Medical Errors and the Management Protocol to be adopted

Minor error is one that presents low risk to the patient and causes no lasting damage. Minor errors should be dealt with methodically and promptly. The patient will expect and deserves courtesy of a truthful explanation of the incident. The explanation should come as soon as possible and by the doctor concerned or a senior colleague. It may be prudent to have a risk management officer present at the interview. The interview may start in an informal manner at the patient's bedside if privacy can be secured or in an interview room and be led by the doctor. The error should be described in non-technical terms. Its management and natural history should be discussed and the implications for the future, if any, be emphasised where appropriate. The discussion should be summarised in the patient's notes. Where the patient does not understand what is going on or is a minor, the next of kin should be present during the interview. If need for a second interview arises, it should take place as soon as possible and the patient should be encouraged to have present such other people as are appropriate. Misinterpretation should be avoided by ensuring good communication. Some minor problems can be dealt with 'in house'. This should not necessarily imply liability or admission. Documentation for the patient to carry as personal record may be useful and relevant to future medical care.

Major error is one that carries high risk to the patient and results in serious effects such as permanent injury or death of the patient. The implications here are grave and warrant the doctor's immediate attention and the full cooperation of his/her team. In this situation, *the protocol to be adopted is in three phases.*

Phase 1

During this phase the doctor must attend to the patient as a matter of priority and summon for assistance as soon as possible, if appropriate.

However, the doctor must remember that every Assistant is a *potential witness* in any future proceedings. Only people capable of contributing to problem-solving should be sought for assistance where possible. The doctor can summon more than one person, but he/she should remember that 'more' is not 'merrier'. In a fatal error, the body becomes the property of the coroner (England and Wales) or the procurator fiscal in (Scotland) in the UK. A senior member of the team should examine the body to *confirm death* and to document any equipment left *in situ*. Documents to be sent to the coroner or the procurator fiscal should be drafted out very carefully and edited by the legal personnel to represent *facts* as opposed to *opinions*. It is at this stage of preparing documents that many mistakes are made.

If the *patient survives* the error, he/she will need appropriate care in a hospital, nursing home, special residential home, or in his/her own home. Hospital care may be in an Intensive Therapy Unit (ITU), also known as Intensive Care Unit (ICU), a High Dependence Unit (HDU), or in an ordinary ward. Subsequent care, therefore, may be in the hands of staff other than those who were involved at the time of the error or adverse event. A detailed handover of the patient is virtually important. It allows for facts of the event to be checked and documented in the presence of the doctor as may be appropriate. During subsequent visits to the patient, the doctor should get updated on the clinical situation of the patient and if possible review all the patient's notes including nursing notes. Any errors should be brought to the attention of the staff and colleagues looking after the patient. Laboratory reports, X-rays, and scan reports should be checked as well.

The original medical records should never be altered, defaced, blotted, covered with correction fluid, or replaced with new written pages. For incomplete entry or errors, appropriate postscripts should be entered, dated, timed, and signed. A line can be drawn through the erroneous part of the notes. The doctor should start a *personal file* of the events in which he/she should include photocopies of the entire medical records of the patient and any personal notes. This personal 'file' will be very vital to any future legal action.

Dealing with *relatives* should be properly approached. It is not easy to communicate with relatives under circumstances of a serious medical error or adverse event. But it must be done and done well at the first opportunity. The doctor must not break bad news on the telephone to the family, except in exceptional circumstances. The telephone can be used to invite relatives into the hospital or surgery for what the caller would say 'important news', and if asked whether there is bad news, the answer should be that the *news is extremely important*. This may prepare the relative(s) for the bad news and allow the doctor to break the bad news in person at a more appropriate place and under more controlled conditions.

Remember the *next patient* if appropriate. The doctor should be concerned for the next patient and avoid exposing such patient to faulty equipment or wrong batch of drugs. All equipment and drugs involved in the occurrence of an error or adverse event should be isolated at once for examination by the experts. Drugs should be checked for batch numbers and expiry dates. After checking, the relevant equipment and suspect drugs should be impounded and locked away if possible. Drugs may be sent away for toxicological studies. Only when all this has been done and completed can the equipment and unused drugs be released for use. The exact routine for checking the equipment should be as recommended by the appropriate manufacturers or academic body. If the checking process reveals an error, the risk manager, a medical defence organisation or legal counsel, should be contacted urgently before committing anything to print. The doctor should keep a copy of the report in his/her personal file. All or part of the medical team involved in the error occurrence or that of the adverse event should be relieved of further duties for a while where possible.

'The show must go on' conformity may lead to yet another disaster. Administrative officials should be made aware of the adverse event as soon as possible, preferably by the doctor concerned or by the most senior member of the team.

Phase 2

The patient who survives the adverse event must remain the doctor's priority. The doctor must see or visit the patient initially on a daily basis and take the opportunity to talk to the relatives present. This may be a difficult role since the patient may be in a very poor state or in a 'persistent vegetative state' (PVS) and a small talk with relatives may be uncomfortable. A substitute but specific person may have to carry out this role and convey the doctor's thoughts to the appropriate people.

The formal interview with relatives needs careful planning as to the place, time, content, and participants. It should take place as soon as possible. It is unacceptable to make relatives wait until the hospital staff find it convenient to break the news. The interview room should be private, spacious, but not large or empty which can be intimidating. Comfortable furniture and 'outgoing only' telephone may be provided. The doctor should never conduct the interview alone. The presence of a colleague will help prevent casual talk but avoid intimidating relatives by the presence of large numbers of staff. The temptation to delegate this responsibility to colleagues who may be more experienced in breaking bad news to relatives (e.g. intensive therapy unit specialists) must be very carefully assessed. For example, a surgeon explaining to patients or relatives an anaesthetic disaster is a recipe for further disaster. Surgeons do not know and need not know the intricacies of the genesis of anaesthetic disasters.

Interview participants should include staff who took part in the management of the patient's adverse event, along with possibly a chaplain or other relevant religious official, a social worker, and if appropriate, an interpreter. If the doctor concerned is a junior member of the team, he/she should ask for a more senior colleague or the head of the department to be present. The team should decide who to be the spokesperson, who should do the introduction, and what should be said. A member of the team who has met the relative(s) in the past, who is an ongoing communicator and one who carries authority in the team, should be selected for this very important position. A support person should be identified as he/she has a very important role to play during this interview. This position is suitable for nursing staff or those trained for such work.

The *introduction* involves welcoming the relatives, confirming their identities, shaking hands with them, and then briefly introducing other persons present and encouraging each other to also shake hands with them. At this point, the introducer may either continue as the spokesperson or hand over to the appointed spokesperson. Breaking the bad news should start with the spokesperson stating regret at having to be the bearer of bad news. He/she should then go straight on to state the worst information first, humanely and truthfully. No attempt should be made to state what happened because precise information will not be absorbed at this time, and the exact details may yet not be apparent. What relatives will remember will be the demeanour of the spokesperson, his/her body language, and actual words said. At this point of the interview, it will be appropriate to temporarily leave the relatives with the designated support person for about ten to fifteen (10-15) minutes' break. The brief departure of most of the team allows a breathing space for the relatives to absorb the impact of what has been said. It also gives the impression of deliberation, courtesy, and respect. Relatives must be allowed to display their grief and be offered sympathy and continued support to be assured. The support person's role while in the room is to listen, comfort, and anticipate common needs such as tissues, telephone, and toilet facilities and to be able to alert the team to special needs. Confrontation is unusual, and relatives deserve the dignity of solitude and time to begin their grieving process. The team may also need that short break to discuss how they felt the information was received, their own responses to the events, and how the interview should continue.

The second part of the interview, after the short break, will start with the team getting back into the interview room, reintroducing themselves, and then allowing the support person to leave the room for a few moments if it seems appropriate. The spokesperson will start the conversation with the expression of personal sorrow at being the bearer of bad news. The interview will then continue with taking the history of the patient or the deceased from relatives. This may be a challenge as this interview will be highly stressful and emotionally charged. Taking a medical history at this time is controversial but may put the doctor on more familiar ground and help establish some dialogue. The history should start at the beginning of the illness or at the time of the accident. Information given to relatives at the time of the patient's admission to hospital should be established and what followed hence thereafter. The story of the illness may be told by the relatives as they understand it. The spokesperson should only assume control of the conversation when there is a total loss of narrative. The vocabulary used by the spokesperson and other team members should avoid use of unnecessary technical terms, and any such terms used should be clarified in appropriate lay terms equivalent.

When the relatives have completed their description, the spokesperson should resume control of the conversation and relate facts as previously agreed by the team. When there is no agreement, then the matter is either omitted or prefaced by a phrase such as 'we are not sure exactly what caused the problem, but we did see that the blood pressure was dropping and the heartbeat became very irregular and then stopped'. The team effort at resuscitation and the sense of team loss should be conveyed to the relatives as it helps to explain the efforts made and the grief shared.

If the patient survived the adverse event, the interview should explain what the current situation is including what treatment is in progress and what to expect at this time of the patient's care. Allow plenty of time for questions from relatives and only conclude the interview when it is apparent that the relatives are fully informed. Those relatives who have not seen the patient should be given the opportunity to do so if they wish. In special areas like the **Intensive Therapy Unit (ITU)**, relatives may be given simple explanations as to the purpose of each machine and tubes connected to the patient. Relatives should be encouraged to speak to the patient, hold hands, and ask questions as they wish.

If the patient dies, relatives should be accompanied by two hospital representatives to ensure that no equipment or material is removed from the body. Once again allow relatives to ask questions. The protocol for procedures at the coroner's or the procurator fiscal's inquest (UK) can be explained at this stage. Allow the family to contact a funeral director to make the necessary arrangements. It is important to stress to the relatives that the matter is out of the hands of the hospital from that stage and that the coroner or the procurator fiscal, as the case may be, is now responsible for ensuring that the correct procedures are followed.

Facts and the interview: The interview should stress facts and not opinions. That the blood pressure dropped is a fact; that there was excessive blood loss is an opinion unless of course the blood loss was measured and exceeded the expected amount of loss. The spokesperson should not imply that it was the patient's fault that he/she came to harm or died. The truth should be told but tactfully. Insults are only a good starting point for a lawsuit. A cover-up will be suspected if a cause given for the disaster is proved incorrect on investigation. It is inappropriate to suggest that nobody knows what went wrong. It is better to explain the facts indicating areas which are to be investigated without speculation or being opinionated about the probabilities of each possible cause.

Avoid incriminating any member of staff directly when the cause of the adverse event is unclear. It is now entirely acceptable for the *doctor to say sorry* and to express regret that an adverse event has occurred. Sorrow expressed in a spontaneous fashion is great comfort to the grieving family, and to do so does not constitute an admission of legal liability. At the end of the interview, arrangements should be made for the welfare of the relatives, and this task may fall on the chaplain or such a person, a social worker, or a member of staff who knows the family well. The family should not be rushed and should get an escort to a convenient exit. This courtesy may be extended by providing a taxi home if the family needs it. When leave is finally taken, do shake hands and give a parting message to the family. A follow-up appointment may be necessary in order to explain the facts as they become known, e.g. after receiving the post-mortem results. This may reduce the aggravation that non-communication can cause.

The referring doctor, if applicable, as well as other specialists who cared for the patient previously, should be informed of what happened to their patient and what is being done. This opens a channel of communication between the doctor concerned and other medical practitioners, and it is also good *etiquette*. Making factual statements concerning the event minimises damage caused by gossip and hearsay and also makes it clear that the doctor involved is not avoiding the issue. This way the doctor may get a chance for 'off the cuff' ventilation of opinions and a chance for identifying unknown prejudices about a particular colleague or institution. As these medical practitioners may be called as witnesses, the doctor concerned should choose his/her words carefully.

The Defusing Session (or Meeting)

This is simply a brief talk from an appropriate principal or leader of the team to recap the events, thank those involved for their assistance, talk about personal feelings resulting from the incident, and to give a 'take away' statement. However, the concept of an 'informal take away' statement is controversial. It is rather a definitive statement than a vacuum of reliable information that will produce an unrecognisable escalating scandal that takes months to die away. If there is an obvious legal threat, those present should be cautioned about careless talk to any outsiders.

The speech should be brief, with tea, coffee, or other beverages being provided. The principal should allow staff to mingle, and the leader should say thank you and inform those present what is being done for the patient and/or relatives. This session also serves as an opportunity to give assurance to the staff that it is normal to be upset at such an adverse result as they have witnessed. The leader indicates how they might feel as normal people who have been through the stress of the day and offers assistance to anyone who feels overwhelmed by the events. Such a leader gauges the need for a formal critical incident stress debriefing (CISD) meeting.

The critical incident stress debriefing (CISD) meeting is best held two to three (2-3) days after the event and should be cleared by a legal counsel. Staff involved with the incident should attend as well as any other particular members of staff from specialties like blood transfusion, laboratory, and operating theatres. Staff whose roles in the hierarchy are totally different and those who do not relate directly with each other should be excluded. Few medical practitioners are at ease in critical incident debriefing meetings with non-medical staff. Regardless of the composition, the format is the same. The head of the department convenes the meeting, and it is run by a trained mental health professional assisted by two peer supporters. Peer supporters are members of the specialty or discipline involved who have had training in the role of peer support. They bridge the perceived gap between the mental health professional and those who are to be debriefed.

Some of the factors determining the need for a critical incident debriefing meeting include a request for such a meeting by some authority, a need for detailed discussion, staff emotional level, and ongoing active media interest in the story. The benefits of such a meeting are improved mental health of the staff involved, better teamwork, reduced resignation rates of staff, and improved productivity. Without a critical incident stress debriefing meeting, the following symptoms may occur among the staff: poor sleeping habits, nightmares, morbid fears of their own families being involved in such an adverse event, altered personal habits, inability to concentrate, low standard of work practices, excessive alcohol consumption, burnout, and post-traumatic stress disorder.

Feelings may run high during the critical incident debriefing meeting. A spate of recent incidents of small children being involved in such incidents or a patient known to the staff or a staff member being a victim would create circumstances under which charged emotions prevail. The meeting should start with a statement of the rules governing such sessions. Such rules include the following:

- *Confidentiality*: No discussion with outsiders is allowed, and no records should be kept by individual members.
- *Performance assessment*: The critical incident stress debriefing meeting should not be used for performance assessment by supervisors.
- *Continuity*: The meeting should be continuous but with personal breaks being allowed to be taken individually with one of the peers accompanying the individual to ensure return. The meeting continues with a round-the-room introduction, every person stating who they are and what their role was on the day of the incident. The meeting goes through the *factual phase* and the *thinking phase*, which leads to the description of the emotional or reaction responses to the problem at hand. Each member describes any symptoms experienced since the incident.

Next comes the *teaching phase* during which the mental health professional teaches what may be expected as normal responses to critical incident stress. This allows members of the group to learn that stress has its problems and sequel.

The *re-entry phase* follows the teaching phase, and here members of the group may ask whatever questions they may have. A summary is then given by the group leader, and the critical incident debriefing meeting is concluded with a reminder that the meeting is entirely confidential. Individuals with particular problems arising from the meeting may stay behind to discuss them with the group leader or with those members of the group more experienced in those matters.

Phase 3

This is the cooling down phase. The doctor should continue to see his/her patient, preferably in person, in a non-fatal incident. If there are problems, the doctor should arrange a meeting with relatives when they visit the patient. Normal conversation about progress of the injured patient will be appropriate. The doctor should not avoid the patient or relatives. In a fatal incident, the family should be informed of the post-mortem results, and this will be the opportunity for a follow-up interview with them. More questions should be expected at that interview.

Doctor's personal record is one of the keys in subsequent legal action. A copy of the *file* should be sent to the appropriate *medical defence organisation*, which will assist in establishing that that report was composed in anticipation of legal action. In most jurisdictions, this will exempt the report from the process of legal discovery (i.e. the requirement to produce documents that may or will be tendered in evidence to support a legal case in the UK). The file should contain photocopies of the medical records of the patient and the personal statement of the events of the incident. Every conceivable detail should be included in the statement. Details of the planned procedure, the date and place, the admitting doctor or consenting doctor, if different, and where appropriate the authority of such doctor should be given in the statement. The duties of the doctor concerned the previous day and on the day of the incident should be stated clearly. The instance when the doctor concerned first became aware of the adverse event and what immediate action was taken should be given in full detail as documented during the event. What was known but not documented during consultation and the implications of the clinical history must be included in the statement. Examination findings and all investigations and their results should be included with any relevant comments by specialists. Also included should be the details of resuscitation, first, by giving a narrative to the documented record, and second, by using information that was not recorded at the time of the incident.

Finally the doctor should print, date and sign the final draft, and either keep it in a safe place or forward it directly to his/her medical defence organisation. This process should be completed within days of the event occurring, long before the formalities of legal action take place.

The Doctor's Mental Health following the occurrence of Medical Error

This may be a topic not much written about. The perceived professional isolation, loss of self-esteem, possible revelation of a chemical (alcohol or drugs) dependency problem, loss of control over events that culminated in the incident, loss of career prospects, potential loss of income, media exposure, and loss of community standing may result in the greatest loss of all—the *suicide* of a *doctor*. This is a devastating permanent answer to a catastrophic but temporary problem. More often, however, failure to work through the event marks the incident as a major psychological stressor which may surface to debilitate the doctor later.

Mechanisms of support for the doctor do vary from place to place and from culture to culture. A *mentor* (someone years older, non-judgemental and non-supervisory; someone able to pass on tips in skills and capable of handling the politics and problems of the doctor's career) should be involved and if possible attend the scene of the incident as soon as it has happened. Together with the head of the department or deputy, the mentor should assist the doctor to complete all the tasks detailed above. A particular individual in the department may have developed the role of being the person the staff turn to for help with their welfare problems. All those around the doctor should recognise the feelings of loss that occur in the situation of a major critical incident. Instead of isolating the doctor, these people should make positive steps to support him/her. Impromptu conversations are useful learning for the listener and a good opportunity for the doctor to ventilate feelings and start grieving for personal 'loss'. This is how humans maintain mental health.

This supportive process should be extended to the doctor's family or next of kin. It is not traditional to make such contact in a major incident, but it is the appropriate thing to do. Good support at home, sympathy, and common purpose will help the healing of the mental scars. This initial communication also opens up a contact channel for the doctor's family who may be the first to recognise that the doctor's mental health has taken a battering. Total change in personal habits, unusual seeking of solitude, irrational displays of temper, and signs of chemical dependence are symptomatic. When it becomes necessary to see a *psychiatrist colleague*, the doctor should expect respect for his/her skills and for his/her intelligence. This professional contact has the added benefit of protection as part of the expected and valued privilege of confidentiality. This, however, may not be absolute in some jurisdictions.

References

1. General Medical Council, Confidentiality: Protecting and Providing Information (Frequently Asked Questions) *GMC Booklet*, April 2004, *www.gmc-uk.org*
2. Janis Smy, The Pitfalls of Breaking Bad News to Patients, *Hospital Doctor*, October 2002, 41, *www.hospital-doctor.net*
3. Helmreich Robert, Error Management: Lessons from Aviation, *British Medical Journal*, *http://bmj.bmjjournals.com/cgi/ijlink*
4. Melanie Hingorani, Tina Wong, et al., Patients' and Doctors' Attitudes to Amount of Information Given after Adverse Events, *British Medical Journal*, **318**, 1999, 640-1.
5. A. R. Aitkenhead, Anaesthetic Disasters: Handling the Aftermath, *Anaesthesia*, **52**, 1997, 477-82.
6. A. Bacon and R. Mason, Cleaning Up Afterwards: Reducing the Threat of Litigation, *Baillère's Clinical Anesthesiology*, **7**(2), 1993, 485-98.
7. William B. Applegate, Physician Management of Patients with Adverse Outcomes, *Arch. Int. Med.*, **146**, 1986, 2249-52.
8. Terry Mizrahi, Managing Medical Mistakes: Ideology, Insularity and Accountability among Internists in Training, *Soc. Sc. Med.*, **19**(2), 1984, 135-46.

Chapter 14

Medical Errors and Litigation: Why do Patients sue Doctors?

Medical manslaughter prosecutions: Between 1867 and 1970, only two (2) doctors were convicted of manslaughter in the UK, although one of them was later pardoned on appeal. A third doctor was acquitted of the charge. Research carried out by Dr Robin Ferner of City Hospital NHS Trust, Birmingham, and published in 2000 showed that during the 1970s and 1980s, only four (4) doctors were charged with manslaughter and seventeen (17) were charged during the 1990s. Another six (6) doctors were tried for manslaughter two and half years after publication of this report.

Conviction rates: Out of twenty one (21) doctors prosecuted for manslaughter between 1970 and 1999, ten (10) were convicted, but three (3) of these had their convictions quashed on appeal. Between 2000 and 2002, out of six (6) doctors charged for manslaughter, only one (1), an anaesthetist, was found guilty of manslaughter and three (3) of the remaining five (5) were acquitted on the direction of the judge. The same judge played a role in the decision to acquit the sixth doctor in this group.

The success rate for medical manslaughter prosecutions is much lower than that of manslaughter generally. The reason is that for the manslaughter charge to stick, it must be proved beyond reasonable doubt that the defendant caused the death. The statistics regarding medical manslaughter prosecutions are different since the early 2000s and interested parties can get up to date information from the Home Office (UK).

The practice of medicine can never be free of errors, and changes are required in the attitudes of both patients and the medical profession with realistic expectations of the limitations of doctors and medicine and greater blame-free openness. Until recently doctors have been reluctant to provide detailed information to patients after the occurrence of medical errors and adverse events, often in an attempt to protect their patients from potentially detrimental anxiety. Doctors may also have been avoiding telling patients because it is a time-consuming, difficult, and unpleasant task. *Telling* patients might result in losing patients' trust or being blamed. In addition, it has been suggested that the current medical culture in which error is often and automatically equated with professional incompetence or inadequacy, such a culture makes admission to either patients or colleagues difficult.

However, it is now accepted that what prompts the overwhelming number of patients to seek *legal advice* about their medical care is failure by doctors and other health care professionals to understand the emotional or human needs of their charges. Most potential litigants turn up at their lawyers' office with little more than a desire to have answers to questions about their care that their doctors could or would not answer. Were it not for the relative inability of some doctors to communicate effectively with their patients, a large percentage of medical litigation would simply never arise, irrespective of the quality of care provided. The real problem therefore is poor communication between doctors and their patients and patients' relatives.

Doctors are at an increased risk for legal and professional sanctions by failing to disclose medical errors and adverse events to their patients. Disclosing errors to patients and patients' relatives, as appropriate, may be the only way doctors can achieve a sense of absolution. However, in the past, there have been no guidelines available to doctors on how to do so. The General Medical Council (UK) revised its guidance on good medical practice, stating that 'after an error or adverse event, a full and honest explanation and an *apology* should be provided to the patient or his/her family, routinely'. In the light of this new regulation, failure to acknowledge a medical error or an adverse event arising during treatment may have serious professional consequences for the doctor concerned. Disclosure may reduce the risk of punitive actions of patients and patients' relatives.

Errors which seriously affect social life, ability to work, and family life or personal relationships are more likely to lead to *litigation*. Intense emotions which continue to be felt for a long time after the injury may also result in patients deciding to take legal action. So the determinants for taking legal action may vary, but the *severity* of the original injury, *insensitive* handling of the event by the doctor and other medical staff concerned, poor or lack of *communication* after the event, unsatisfactory or *dishonest* explanations, and lack of *apology* are very important factors which can greatly increase the risk of litigious intentions of patients and their relatives.

After an error or adverse event, patients want not only the disclosure of the event but also an admission of responsibility and details of how the event will be managed and its long-term effects. Patients seek greater honesty, an appreciation of the severity of the injuries suffered, and assurances that lessons have been learnt. Some patients and their relatives may take legal action because they are concerned with the *standards of care* provided and want to prevent similar incidents happening in the future. Patients may want an explanation as to how and why the incident happened in the first place. *Accountability*, a belief that staff or an organisation should have to account for actions or inactions, and a desire to punish the offender, may yet be another motive in litigation. Finally, the injured patients and their relatives may seek *compensation* for actual losses, for pain and suffering, and for care to be provided in future for their family and dependants. If litigation is viewed solely as a legal and financial problem, many fundamental issues will be neither addressed effectively nor resolved. A no-fault compensation system, currently operational in some countries, however well intended, will not address all patients' concerns and those of their relatives. So it seems controversial.

Medical Boards and Law Courts in the UK and USA

Fidelity is an integral part of the doctor-patient relationship. This calls for open and honest communication even about very difficult processes. Medical ethics calls for doctors to tell their patients of errors and adverse events when they occur 'if such information significantly affects the care of such patients'. The challenge, of course, is how to communicate such information to their patients. This has been discussed in previous sections of this book. Involvement of the courts and disciplinary bodies is an increasingly common phenomenon in today's medical practice, and although the usual outcome is favourable to the doctor, the price of success is still very high.

A majority of the world's legal systems stem from the *British* legal system. The *USA* operates largely similar systems in its various states. More 'malpractice' suits have been filed in the USA than in all other countries combined. In the USA, the *contingency fee* has been the driving force behind this trend and accounts for between 35 per cent and 50 per cent of *awards* given to injured parties. The emphasis has been on awarding *damages* rather than *how* and *why* the malpractices were committed. All malpractice cases going to court in the USA involve *jury trials*. The high awards and frequency of cases going to court led to a practice of what the medical profession called 'defensive medicine', and a demand for higher insurance premiums followed. Some states in the USA introduced restrictions on the amount of damages to be awarded, the level of contingency fees, and the awarding of costs against plaintiffs with frivolous claims.

Medical Disciplinary Boards in the UK

Disciplinary medical boards in the UK fall into two categories:

Government or State Authorised Registration Boards: The *General Medical Council* (GMC) has the power to register or license doctors and dentists. The *disciplinary board* of the employing authority is known as the *employer disciplinary board*.

Registration boards usually allow legal representation during the hearing of cases brought before them, and employer-based boards normally do not allow such representation unless dismissal is on the cards. Advice from the appropriate legal counsel can greatly assist the preparation for an appearance before the employer disciplinary board.

The National Health Service (NHS) Indemnity Scheme (UK)

The *indemnity scheme* was introduced in January 1990 to cover NHS hospitals and primary care staff, excluding general practitioners (GPs). However, it was advisable for all registered doctors to continue to be members of medical defence organisations for continuing advice and assistance regarding medical-legal issues and other areas of medical practice not covered under the scheme. Crown indemnity arrangements for medical practitioners in the Ministry of Defence (MoD) were introduced at the same time with broad provisions. Responsibility for the indemnity scheme was given to what were then district health authorities (under the terms of Health Circular 89: 34: DoH 1989), and this was passed on to their successors, the *NHS trusts* and *NHS trust foundations*, who were instructed to 'assume responsibility for new and existing claims of medical negligence'. Medical staff were relieved of their contractual requirement to belong to a defence organisations. This change in responsibility meant that the essential decisions about handling claims and the defence or settlement thereof devolved on the trust chief executives, usually on the basis of independent expert medical opinion and using the trusts' own legal advisors. Because of the exclusive nature of the process, these legal advisors became de facto legal advisors of the doctors concerned, and it became entirely right and proper for employees and ex-employees to cooperate fully with them and with the managers when a claim had to be investigated.

There are three important factors which did not alter with the introduction of the NHS indemnity scheme. These are as follows:

1. The *civil law* and the need to establish negligence and causation.
2. The moral responsibility of health authorities, NHS trusts, and trust foundations to compensate patients who suffer through medical negligence.
3. The moral responsibility of health authorities, NHS trusts, and trust foundations to uphold the *good standing* of medical practitioners in their employment when negligence cannot be established.

One particular important implication of the NHS indemnity scheme, which caused concern among doctors, was addressed by the Department of Health when it instructed NHS trusts about potential settlements. The instruction was that 'in deciding whether to resist a claim or seek out-of-court settlement, Health Authorities and those advising them, should pay particular attention to any *view* which is expressed by the *medical practitioner concerned* and any potentially damaging effect on the professional reputation of such a practitioner. Health authorities should also have clear regard to any point of principle of wider implications raised by the case and the cost involved'. It is worth pointing out that defending the medical practitioner was not part of the remit of the scheme and the NHS indemnity scheme does not cover every medico-legal eventuality.

Medical defence organisations no longer influence the outcome of hospital-based claims in the way they once did. The GMC's booklet *Duties of a Doctor* (1998) specifically instructed medical practitioners thus, 'In your interests and those of patients, doctors should have professional indemnity cover for any part of their work not covered by their employer's indemnity scheme'. Medical defence organisations in UK use their own database of medical negligence claims to produce reports drawing the attention of their members to areas of risk in their own specialties.

Clinical Negligence Scheme for NHS Trusts (CNST) in the UK

A *national health trust litigation authority* was established in April 1989 to deal with all negligence cases arising in the NHS trusts. This body took over the trust-funded clinical negligence scheme for trusts. Its emphasis was on settling cases faster, fairly, and with minimal or no bureaucracy. It sets standards for the NHS trusts and underwrites their legal claims in England and Wales. It postulates that in cases of serious adverse outcomes, patients will be entitled to a full explanation of what happened. Procedures should be in place to encourage openness and for patients to be given as much information as they require and to implement early release of medical records and early settlement of claims. An average medical negligence claim was taking five years, on average, to resolve, and some claims have been known to drag on for much longer than this.

Pre-action Protocol in resolving Clinical Disputes

The 'pre-action' *protocol* for the resolution of clinical disputes, which was the first major project of the Clinical Disputes Forum set up way back in 1996, laid down the steps that both parties would have to take from the moment a patient first raises concerns about medical care and treatment. The 'pre-action' protocol encouraged greater openness and minimisation of the atmosphere of mistrust and tendency to sue. It also encouraged, where appropriate, quicker resolution of cases without litigation. This protocol became part of the 'new' *court rules* for the revamped civil justice system.

The courts expected the protocol to be observed by everyone involved in a claim, and they would impose penalties for non-compliance. A patient starting legal action without giving the health-care trust involved enough time to offer redress could be penalised by cost-order, and a health-care trust that delays in handing over patients' medical records and related information could be refused more time to file a defence.

Common Law of Confidence as applicable to Doctors

The law on *confidentiality* known as common law in the UK requires *consent* for disclosure of identifiable data unless there is a legal provision authorising or requiring disclosure of such data or there is an overriding public interest in the disclosure of such data.

Disclosure in relation to a court order: the courts, both civil and criminal, have powers, by virtue of the various pieces of legislation that govern their operation, to order disclosure of information. A court order will generally explain the basis on which disclosure is being ordered.

Complaints, Claims, and their Management

A *complaint* is defined as 'an expression of dissatisfaction or concern, in verbal or written form, which may be made by a user of the service or his/her advocate'. All complaints received must be recorded by the person receiving them and the patient liaison department must receive a copy as soon as possible. All responses to the complaint must be recorded, including an indication of whether or not the complainant is satisfied with the outcome of his/her complaint. All correspondence on complaints must be kept separately from clinical records. Resolving complaints at source (i.e. local resolution) must be the primary aim, and all complaints must be taken seriously. Complainants must be assured that their complaints will be treated in confidence and with sensitivity. The *Independent Review Panel convener* may handle cases where complainants are dissatisfied with results from the local resolution process. The Health Service Commissioner or the *Ombudsman*, in UK, may deal with some complaints which fail to be resolved by the Independent Review Panel.

References

1. Clare Dyer: Supreme Court abolishes immunity for Expert Witnesses. British Medical Journal 2011: **342**: 785.
2. Dr Patrick Hoyte, Complaints to the GMC: Non-clinical, Health and Performance, *MDU Journal*, **19**, 2003, 22-5.
3. Francesca Robinson, Doctors Behind Bars, *Hospital Doctor*, May 2003, 24-6, *www.hospital-doctor.net*
4. Clare Dyer, Doctors Face Trial for Manslaughter As Criminal Charges Against Doctors Continue to Rise, *British Medical Journal*, **325**, 2002, 63.
5. Merry, et al., Errors, Medicine, and the Law, *British Medical Journal*, **324**, 2002, 304.
6. Merry, et al., *British Medical Journal*, 2002, 649-50.
7. Shain Marr, NHS Redress Scheme for Clinical Negligence: Making Amends, *www.dh.gov.uk/CMO*
8. Clare Dyer, Junior Doctor Charged with Manslaughter after Medical Error, *British Medical Journal*, **325**, 2002, 616.
9. Editorial (Prosecuting doctors over errors is not the answer), *Hospital Doctor*, July 2002, 14, *www.hospital-doctor.net*
10. John Camm, Risk of Litigation on the Rise, *Hospital Doctor*, August 2000, 10.
11. Martin Hutchinson, GMC Votes for Revalidation, *Hospital Doctor* (UK), December 1999, 1.
12. Dr Gamal Hammand, Communication Vital, *Hospital Doctor* (UK), December 1999, 22.
13. P. Hoyte, Understanding NHS Indemnity, *Hospital Medicine*, **9**, 1998, 726-7.

Chapter 15

The process of Litigation in the Medical profession in UK and USA

Civil actions occur when a patient or his/her relatives *sue* under the *law of negligence*, here called *litigation*. If something goes wrong and the patient is harmed or dies, one could be called to account for one's actions or inactions under the *law of negligence*, although under the doctrine of vicarious liability, it may be the employer who is pursued by the patient's lawyer in the knowledge that, if successful, the employer would be able to meet the compensation awarded. If the patient was harmed due to one's partial or total negligence, such patient or his/her relatives could, in theory, sue that individual doctor.

There are two major differences among the *American*, *UK*, and *other* countries' medical litigation forums. They are the *contingency fees* and the *jury trials*, as already mentioned in the book. Otherwise, American civil courts are quite similar to those found in other parts of the world. Procedural variations occur but under the same principle that the injured person must prove that the doctor or an institution breached the standard of care and caused harm. Before the trial or hearing, each side 'discovers' information from the other side. Usually this involves a *deposition* of the parties plus *disclosures* of the identity and opinions of all expert witnesses. All documents and other demonstrative evidence must be revealed before the trial. A mistake here may lose the case even before the trial has begun.

Meeting with the Solicitor (or Attorney in USA): The doctor's first contact with *litigation* may be by a letter or telephone call from a solicitor or in the

USA the attorney who his/her defence organisation or insurance company has selected to represent him/her. If the same solicitor is representing the doctor's employer or related institution, as it may happen under the NHS indemnity scheme, there is potential for conflict of interest because there is more than one client involved. In the USA, the doctor may first meet with an assistant attorney or an associate of the trial attorney, but in the UK and in those countries using British-based legal system, a solicitor will initially handle the case before briefing a barrister, as the case may be.

The doctor or professional involved and his/her solicitor must develop a proper understanding of each other from the start. There must be total trust between them from the beginning if problems are to be minimised. The doctor should not direct at the solicitor the hostility, anger, and displeasure at being sued. It is the solicitor's job to ask the doctor direct, detailed, and sometimes painful questions regarding the doctor's explanations for performing or not performing certain procedures. Some enquiries may even sound accusatory, and the doctor may feel that the solicitor is indulging in a cross-examination. The doctor should not take the questions personally because the solicitor is merely trying to examine the case from three perspectives: the adversary, the doctor, and the judge and jurors. Personal feelings and pride must be forsaken if the solicitor and the doctor are to work together effectively to win the case.

The Courts: Which Court?

In the UK, there are *coronial* and *procurator fiscal* courts at which a coroner presides and *civil* and *criminal* courts at which *judges* preside with a *jury*.

The Coroner's Court

This court enquires into deaths where there is a possibility of unnatural cause of death or when a doctor cannot issue a death certificate. The court seeks to provide an explanation as to what occurred. It does not award damages but may refer cases to the other courts. Evidence submitted in this court may not be admissible in the other courts. The proceedings in a coroner's court are called an *inquest*. Before the inquest takes place, the doctor concerned with the case is required to submit a statement which could contain a factual account of the events. This statement must be written in the first person and be based on available medical records. No opinions should be expressed. Sometimes a more senior doctor may be asked to provide a report to the coroner on behalf of all those involved in the incident or management of the patient before death. This report too should be factual and identify who did what so that the coroner can decide who should be called to give evidence at the inquest. In some circumstances, interests of the hospital or such employer and those of the doctor may diverge, but proper legal advice may address this problem.

The Civil Court

This is where the action is. Legal actions start in the same courts as criminal cases, but here the government or state only provides the forum. The government does not prosecute. A plaintiff initiates a civil action alleging that the doctor or hospital authority departed from the standard of care, a standard generally defined as 'what a reasonably competent medical practitioner or provider would do under the same circumstances or similarly, a standard expected from the hospital'. The plaintiff may claim malpractice, lack of 'informed consent', or a breach of contract. All these situations do involve a standard of care.

The Criminal Court:

A criminal court works on the principle that the government or state, generally as a result of police investigations, seeks the prosecution of an individual or an institution because of an alleged breach of a criminal code. The presumption of innocence applies and the government's proof required is high. A criminal court may be a magistrate's court, a county court, a circuit court, or Supreme Court. The lower courts may hear the initial charges in major proceedings but then refer the cases to higher courts for a full trial. In the USA, trial courts handle all criminal cases first, and then appeals are based entirely on the records made in the lower courts. Recent reports point to there being more cases of criminal prosecution than traditional civil actions. In the UK, investigations by police may take several months to years to complete, a problem not yet resolved.

If a doctor is approached by police during such investigations, he/she should first contact a medical defence organisation immediately before responding to police enquiries. Under no circumstances should a written statement be submitted to the police, particularly under *caution*, without legal advice. Police investigations may result in no action being taken or the case being referred to the Crown Prosecution Service (CPS), which, in turn, may decide not to take any action or may decide to prosecute. The medical defence organisations are invariable source of support and encouragement in these matters, and membership is more than worthwhile.

Meeting the Solicitor (or Attorney in USA)

Discussions with the solicitor are protected by the *lawyer-lawyer-client privilege* and therefore are completely confidential. This privilege, however, extends only to between the lawyer, his/her agents, and the doctor. Hence, the legal view is that the doctor should avoid discussing the case with anyone else but the solicitor. The doctor must be completely frank with the solicitor, admitting any errors made and problems that might have arisen during clinical management of the patient. The doctor must divulge to the solicitor every fact, detail, and thoughts related to the incident. Knowledge of a potentially negligent act early on in the process will increase the solicitor's chances of curing or at least minimising its effect on the outcome of the case. An eleventh-hour confession gives the solicitor no time to adequately defend the doctor and almost certainly causes irreparable damage to the case.

Medical Records tendered to the Legal Team

The doctor must obtain a full, legible copy of all records regarding the patient's care at the earliest opportunity. These records should include records of the patient's treatment before and after the event. They may direct attention to the pertinent areas to investigate for additional preparation and examination. The doctor should become familiar with every entry in all the medical records. The more knowledgeable he/she is about these records, the more credible is the testimony at the trial. However, the doctor should remember that for tactical reasons his/her solicitor may not want him/her to be too knowledgeable about alleged consequences of the incident before *deposition*.

Discovery Process

This is the process whereby the parties and their solicitors attempt to uncover, review, and evaluate all the evidence having any bearing on the facts of the case. Few civil malpractice cases proceed to trial or hearing without engaging in a process called *discovery*. The discovery process occurs after the plaintiff has filed a lawsuit and before the trial begins. Solicitors may employ various *discovery techniques* during the course of the lawsuit, such as written questions called *interrogatories*, distribution of *documents* and *other non-oral evidence*, and *depositions*.

Depositions

Depositions are the most important tool of *discovery* in a medical malpractice case. It is an out-of-court testimony of a witness recorded in writing under *oath* or under *affirmation*. It is intended for use in a lawsuit. In the USA, a court reporter records the attorney's questions, and the witness answers them and later prepares a written transcript. Lawyers, the defendant, and plaintiff are usually present. Depositions are less formal than the court proceedings, and they typically take place in one of the lawyers' offices. No judge is present, and *evidentiary rules* are relaxed. The doctor and his counsel must assume that they are in a courtroom because anything said under oath at deposition becomes part of the official record of the lawsuit and may be introduced as evidence at trial. The doctor should receive a copy of the *deposition transcript* and check it for any errors or wrong spellings. If the case goes to court, reviewing the transcript will aid the doctor in repeating, in the witness box, much of what has been said at the deposition, which exhibits consistency. After the deposition, the doctor must keep involved in the case and ask his/her lawyer to update him/her and pass on copies of all correspondence and legal papers.

The Adjudicatory Hearing

All the pre-trial activity is in preparation for the *adjudicatory hearing*. The doctor needs to prepare for this even more thoroughly than for the deposition. He/she must painstakingly review the medical records and rehearse the proposed testimony. Mock cross-examination now becomes a necessity. If the doctor has no experience in malpractice case proceedings in court, he/she should take every chance to visit the court and watch a case in progress. The doctor must attend court every day of the trial and be assured that the plaintiff will also be there. In court, the doctor should present a clean and tidy appearance but should dress conservatively. Overdressing will make him appear overly prosperous to the *fact finder* in contrast to the poor wronged plaintiff. A hard-working professional should be seen to be oblivious of the trappings of success.

The most important goal to achieve at the trial is *credibility*. This is achieved by somebody who considers and responds to the questions asked in a clear and straightforward manner. Jargon and highly technical terms are better avoided during *testimony*, thereby escaping the appearance of the unfeeling technician. If the doctor does not understand a question, he/she should say so to the *fact finder*. He/she should never risk appearing non-responsive to a question and should not volunteer unsolicited information. A doctor will be more persuasive if courteous and non-adversarial to the opposing counsel and plaintiff. As in deposition, the plaintiff's lawyer may try to mischaracterise the doctor's testimony or do other things to intimidate him/her. The doctor must avoid becoming angry, rattled, or hesitant under such pressure because these are precisely the reactions the opposing counsel seeks to elicit. So the appropriate response is to remain composed. Above all, the doctor must tell the truth, for failure to do so would be both morally wrong and may constitute perjury.

Expert Witness

The Expert Witness Institute (EWI) was established in 1996 as an umbrella organisation for all expert witnesses. The British Medical Association (BMA) was a founding sponsor of the institute but later withdrew from it. There is a Register, and entry to it is essential for those who wish to engage in medico-legal activity in the UK.

An Expert Witness forms a critical part of the medical malpractice litigation team. The law requires that the *plaintiff's lawyer* proves, usually through expert testimony, that the *defendant* violated the applicable standard of care in treating the patient concerned. Correspondingly, the doctor will have an expert who testifies to his/her compliance with standards of care, the appropriateness of decisions made and actions taken, and perhaps the inevitability of the patient's outcome, even with the best of care. The *fact finder* then determines whether the treatment constituted negligence, based largely on the expert witness's testimony.

It is important to remember that the *fact finder* usually considers the expert witness more objective than the parties. Consequently the doctor and his/her lawyer should take great care in the selection of their expert witness. Possession of some extraordinary reputation and personal character beyond reproach would make an expert witness very valuable. The expert witness must have unusual knowledge and background in his/her particular medical specialty. He/she must possess an impressive demeanour and come across as a self-confident individual who is fully versed in all aspects of the case with the ability to make a poised presentation before the *fact finder* overrides credentials. The expert witness must know the facts perfectly well because a witness who forgets the name of the patient, key dates and times, or events in the case will hardly impress the *fact finder*. The expert witness must be honest in the intellectual interpretation and evaluation of the facts and at least appear impartial. An expert who exhibits integrity will gain respect and support of the *fact finder* and will be the one who is believed.

A guide book *Medical Experts, What We Expect From You*, prepared by a firm of lawyers in the UK, is available, and many medical experts have found it extremely useful.

Civil Justice System in England and Wales, UK

The civil justice system in England and Wales was changed following a review by Lord Woolf in 1994. The aims of the review were to improve access to justice and to reduce the costs of litigation. Previously there had been an escalating cost of expert witnesses and delays caused by the need to engage these experts. The report expressed concern at the way expert witnesses had become partisan advocates rather than neutral givers of professionally based opinions. The basic premise of the rules is that the expert's function is to help the court, not to advance the case of the side by whom the expert is paid. Expert testimony is to help the courts to ascertain what is accepted and the proper practice in specific cases, ensuring that professionally generated standards from real clinical situations are generally applied rather than standards enunciated in rhetoric of clinical guidelines.

Four areas of clinical expert's practice were to change following *Lord Woolf's* review:

- *The first area of change* was that clinical experts were to increasingly be appointed, not by one side or the other but jointly, either with both parties' agreement or at the discretion of the court. Such an expert was to play a neutral role in the proceedings. However, the new rules made provision for both sides in a medical negligence action to use their own experts.
- *The second area of change* was the standardisation of the clinical content in the reports prepared for the courts. Clinicians, for instance, were to set out not only their professional views but also those of any other 'relevant recognised body of opinion'. This was to make medico-legal reports not only well referenced but also longer and more demanding on the expert witness.
- *The third area of change* was the reduction in the volume of work available to medical expert witnesses. Expert evidence was to be received by the courts if it was reasonably essential to resolve the issue before the courts. Most evidence was to be put to the courts in writing, making oral evidence from the experts the exception rather than the rule.
- *The fourth area of change* was that the amount of *fees* for medico-legal work was to be reduced. The fees would only be allowed by the courts if they were in proportion to the value of the claim. The rules allowed the courts to limit the amount of fees that the expert witnesses were to be paid.

Doctors and medical-legal skilled lawyers should have one common objective—that of improving health care. This common interest should bind both professions in what could be a happy alliance. Increased understanding between both professions of the root causes of medico-legal claims is vital if inroads in improving health care and reducing claims are to be successful. Medicine is much at risk from inept lawyers as from inept doctors, and doctors share equal responsibility with lawyers in the search for understanding.

Courts and Clinical Guidelines: Courts may not adopt standards of care advocated in clinical guidelines as legal 'gold standards' because the mere fact that a guideline exists does not in itself establish that compliance with it is reasonable in the circumstances or that non-compliance is negligent. Clinical guidelines can only assist the doctor, but they cannot be used to mandate, authorise, or outlaw treatment options.

References

1. Clare Dyer: Supreme Court abolishes immunity for Expert Witnesses. British Medical Journal 2011: **342**: 785.
2. Troyen Brennan, Colin M. Sox, et al., Relation Between Negligent Adverse Events and the Outcome of Medical Malpractice Litigation. The New England Journal of Medicine, 335, 1996(26),1963-67.
3. Dr Gemmell, Prof. R. Mahajan, Advancing Patient Safety, *Bulletin: Royal College of Anaesthetists*, **51**, 2008, 2625.
4. Dr John Gilberthorpe, Reforms to the Coroners' Service, *MDU Journal*, **19**, 2003, 3.
5. Editorial (Jailing doctors for their errors is not the answer), *Hospital Doctor*, December 2003, 16.
6. Dr Matthew Robson, Behind the Scenes: the Life of a Claim, *MDU Journal*, **19**, 2003, 8-10.
7. Mark Friston, New Rules for Expert Witnesses, *British Medical Journal*, **318**, 1999, 1365.
8. Melanie Hingorani, Tina Wong, et al., Patients and Doctors' Attitudes to Amount of Information Given after Adverse Events, *British Medical Journal*, **318**, 1999, 640-1.
9. Prof. Daniel Simons, Medical Negligence Claims, *MDU Journal*, 1999, **15**, 11-12.
10. Freeth Cartwrite/Hunt Dickins Solicitors, Medical Experts: What We Expect from You, *CME Bulletin*, **2**(1), 1998.
11. Dr Patrick Hoyte, National Health Service Indemnity Scheme, *Hospital Medicine*, **59**, 1998, 9.
12. A. R. Aitkenhead, Anaesthetic Disasters: Handling the Aftermath, *Anaesthesia*, **52**, 1997, 477-82.

13. A. B. Witman, Deric Park, et al., How Do Patients Want Physicians to Handle Mistakes? *Arch. Intern. Med.*, **156**, 1996, 2565-9.
14. Charles Vincent, Magi Young, et al., Why Do People Sue Physicians? *The Lancet*, **343**, 1994, 1609-13.
15. William B. Applegate, Physician Management of Patients with Adverse Outcomes, *Arch. Intern. Med.*, **146**, 1986, 2249-52.

Chapter 16

Reducing the occurrence of
Medical Errors and Adverse Events

The American Medical Association (AMA) started a *medical error-reduction initiative* (MERI) in 1996 and established National Patient Safety Foundation (NPSF), which was based in Chicago. This was the result of *a coalition* of organisations including the *National Council on Patient Information and Education* (*NCPIE), drug companies*; and *Kaiser Permanent Health Maintenance Organisation*. The *coalition goals* were the improvement of medical management of patients, education of patients, and treatment outcomes. This was to be achieved by identifying barriers to sound clinical practices in ambulatory health-care settings as well as in office practice. The National Patient Safety Foundation was to fund research on identification and prevention of human and organisational errors. There was also the *Institute for Safe Medical Practice*, which worked together with the *U.S. pharmacopoeia* on the medical errors reporting programme. Doctors were to call this institute and report errors or potential errors (near misses) with medications and medical devices anonymously. The most fundamental change that was needed, if medical institutions were to make meaningful progress in error reduction and error prevention, was a cultural one. Doctors had to accept the notion that error is an accompaniment of the human condition, even among the conscientious professionals with high standards of medical practice. Errors must be accepted as evidence of system flaws, not character flaws. It should be remembered that not every *injury* or *mistake* is necessarily the result of an error. It may be the result of a system or process that was inappropriate to begin with.

Occupational Health Service and Medical Errors

Occupational Health Service in medical institutions has increasingly been recognised as very useful because it addresses particular employee problems as well as investigates broader problems affecting several employees in an organisation. The service addresses the need for *stress reduction* and *stress management* at the workplace. It provides psychotherapy management training, establishes support groups, and offers confidential non-judgemental counselling service, all of which are important in managing stress at the workplace. External changes in lifestyle and working environment, as well as internal changes in behaviour, perception, and biological response, are essential. The main strategies for reducing work-related stress involves optimising the workplace with the help of the occupational health specialist now called the *consultant occupational physician* and balancing work stress with a healthy lifestyle which includes relaxing activities, a change in personal and work attitude, and behaviour where necessary, always starting with small changes. A consultant occupational physician is of great help to underperforming doctors and other staff. He/she acts as an independent advisor on any contributory health problems and ensures that appropriate action and support is provided for the failing doctor. Such a consultant facilitates specialist referrals, coordinates graded return-to-work programmes, and as a last option, supports an application for ill-health retirement. It is important to take away the feelings of stigma and failure that often obsess people with stress symptoms and which lead to an increase in their pressure levels.

Clinical Governance in the National Health Service (NHS), UK

There are many definitions of clinical governance, one of which was given in the earlier chapters of this book. Other definitions are as follows:

- *Clinical Governance* is 'a framework through which the National Health Service organisations are accountable for continuously improving the quality of their services and safeguarding high standards of health care by creating an environment in which excellence in clinical care will flourish'.

- *The Department of Health* (DoH) defined clinical governance as 'the process by which each part of the NHS quality-assures its clinical decisions'.

Backed by a statutory duty of quality, clinical governance introduced a system of continuous improvement in health care in the NHS.

a) *Clinicians* would probably define clinical governance as 'the acceptance of responsibility of individual doctors to work in a way which is consistent with the values and strategic objectives of the organisation in which they are employed'.
b) *The General Medical Council (GMC)* defined clinical governance as 'a process whereby specialists re-affirm their on-going performance in order to keep their place on the medical register'.

Clinical governance was introduced with the publication of a government white paper called 'The New NHS Modern: Dependable' in December 1997. In broad terms, the government wanted to introduce quality assurance in health care, and clinical governance was part of it. This concept was expanded in another government paper called 'A First Class Service: Quality in the NHS' published in 1998, the salient point of which was that the government started a ten-year modernisation programme to ensure fair access to prompt high-quality health care whenever and wherever a patient was treated in the NHS. A number of government bodies were introduced to monitor and promote high-quality health care.

The National Institute for Clinical Excellence (NICE) was introduced on 1April 1999 and provided a single focus for clear, consistent guidance for clinicians about which treatments work best for which patients. NICE set out common standards in England and Wales for the treatment of particular conditions and the appropriate use of new and existing health-care technologies. The Commission for Health Improvement (CHI), now called Quality Assurance Agency (QAA), was set up by the government for the independent assessment of local activities aimed at improving the quality of health care. It inspects local clinical governance arrangements.

Clinical governance sets out a comprehensive framework for improving quality and not just managing poor performance, encompassing everything from audit, self-regulation to lifelong learning. All these elements of clinical governance, namely, audit, self-regulation, and lifelong learning are interdependent, and one should not be implemented without the other. Clinical governance can pick out the failing doctors as well as raise overall clinical standards. It endeavours to help failing doctors improve their standards.

National Patient Safety Agency (NPSA) in England and Wales, UK

The National Patient Safety Agency was established in July 2003. It was created to oversee a new national reporting and learning system (NRLS) for adverse events and near misses and to learn lessons and improve patients' safety across the NHS. It promotes an open and fair culture that encourages the staff to anonymously report incidents and near misses through the national reporting system. Patients and carers were also encouraged to report incidents. In a document 'Organisation with a Memory', the agency was given some specific targets as reproduced below:

- Reduce to zero the number of patients dying or being paralysed by maladministered spinal injections by 2001 (yet to be met).
- Reduce by 25 per cent the number of instances of harm in the field of obstetrics and gynaecology which result in litigation by 2005.
- Reduce by 40 per cent the number of serious errors in the use of prescribed drugs by 2005.
- Reduce to zero the number of suicides by mental health patients as a result of hanging from non-collapsible beds or shower curtain rails on wards by 2005.

The agency now has a rapid response reporting (RRR) system which issues alerts to medical staff about new or under-recognised risks. The trigger of an RRR is reported deaths or serious events that may be seen as 'one off' by local organisations but which the agency, looking at them at a national level, recognises as system weaknesses for which fixes are available to benefit all NHS trusts. All organisations are required to act on these alerts within a given time, and compliance is monitored by regulators. The process of generating RRRs is driven by patient-safety incidents reported by health care staff. It is, today, one of the largest and most comprehensive reporting systems in the world.

The NPSA has these websites: (*www.nrls.npsa.nhs.uk/resources/type/alerts/.* and *www.npsa.org.uk*) for up to date information on its services.

Continuing Professional Development (CPD) in the UK

Doctors continue to learn through different ways in their professional careers. They live and practice in a rich learning environment, and they are constantly involved in professional interaction, conversation, educational meetings, and seminars, usually with good feedback. The learning process, however, is a complex one. Multiple continuing professional development interventions targeted at specific behaviour can lead to a positive change in that behaviour. The system of managed continuing professional development encourages targeted educational activities where appropriate. Research, on the other hand, seems to suggest that education is not a strong factor in changing clinicians' behaviour at all. Where education has an effect is through medical journals, scientific meetings, and seminars which are cited as the most effective. Doctors' learning is integrated with their practice. The style of integrated practice and learning develops during the successive stages of medical education. Such learning through practice is called 'situated learning'.

Doctors must keep up to date with a rapidly changing knowledge base and be accountable to their patients and the rest of the public for the standards and modernity of the health care they provide. So providing opportunities for learning and making provision for proper assessment of learning needs is an essential part of continuing professional development planning. Active approaches to learning based on adult learning theory are advocated by some, whether or not their value is proven for doctors. There is no 'best' method of learning for doctors. The key to effective continuing professional development is how it is managed, not in the method by which it is undertaken.

Professional learning methods used by doctors can be grouped as follows:

Academic Activities: *meetings* and *conferences*; learning from *managed quality processes*; learning from *special events and workshops;* and learning from peer-led discussion of *clinical incidents.*

Some Royal colleges in the UK may not officially recognise some of the ways in which doctors continue to learn and develop simply because a number of these programmes are difficult to monitor in terms of the hours spent. However, these are part of the learning environment of every doctor in the country and therefore must be recognised and valued within any system of managed continuing professional development for each doctor rather than only the monitory, quantifiable events of learning.

In Europe, continuing professional development is largely a professionally driven activity based on medical activities for a set number of hours a year, unlike in the UK where organisers of educational activities are allocated certified medical education (CME) points for participants. Although there has been some unease about the vast 'CME industry', there is some evidence that well-crafted, well-targeted CME programmes do improve not only doctors' performance but also health-care outcomes. CME programmes are becoming more innovative, international, and relevant to patient care, and it would appear the dream for the future is certified medical education.

The way forward is for the providers and consumers to recognise their professional obligations and to commit themselves to effective evidence-based continuing medical education. Periodic revalidation is being introduced in the UK and in a number of other countries. The challenge is to find ways of monitoring the competences expected of doctors in the future while bearing in mind the wise advice offered by W. B. Cameron in 1963 that 'not everything that counts can be counted, and not everything that can be counted, counts'.

In the USA, similar programmes called 'recertification programmes' use *examinations* and *performance assessments* as 'snapshots' of competence and are taken every seven (7) to ten (10) years. In other countries, most programmes evaluate documented participation in continuing medical education as evidence of continuing medical competence of their medical specialists. Some CME programmes use Internet to document self-directed learning from practice and to monitor performance.

Philip Bashook and Parboosingh summarised their study on recertification (published in *British Medical Journal*, **316**, 1998, 545-8) by asserting that recertification should assess real performance in practice and competence to continue to learn.

Medical Ethics and Medical Errors

Ethical issues are everywhere in medicine. Patients have in the past been used as teaching 'objects' without being fully informed and consented. Terminal diagnoses have routinely been withheld from patients, and the mentally ill have been drugged before any consent has been sought. Some expensive treatments may not be available to certain patients even today. There may be reasonable counter arguments to these assertions, of course, and some of the objections may be important to individuals. Some doctors, for instance, may feel offended by the introduction of a formal ethics scheme because they feel their practice is ethical enough.

Most doctors are aware of *ethical oaths* and *principles*, but codes and standards are only a starting point for practical morality. Codes cannot tell doctors how to interpret their clauses and declarations or how to apply principles intelligently in situations that require balanced judgement. For this, it would appear that ethical analysis is essential. Ethical analysis is a craft that requires intellectual stamina, the knowledge of moral theory, the understanding of the purposes of health care, and a good practical grasp of everything relevant to a case in hand. Ethical reasoning is an essential component in professional staff development and should improve patient safety and public confidence. It is a useful tool in risk management, and by increasing patient satisfaction, litigation can be reduced. A doctor proving his/her competence to colleagues is the ethical pathway to future career progression. Blind faith is out, and consumer choice is in.

Medical ethics is an all-encompassing specialty tackling dilemmas from the start of life to after death. One strand which runs through all these and has changed most is that of *communication*. Blind trust in doctors and beneficent paternalism towards patients are out, and informed choice and consumer involvement are in. Until the recent past, doctors assumed patients would get upset if informed of a serious diagnosis like cancer. It was assumed that patients did not want to know what they were suffering from. However, we have now made very significant improvement in this attitude. A *Scottish Study*, in 1996, showed that *96 per cent* of patients attending a cancer centre specifically wanted to know if their illness was cancer and *76 per cent* of the patients wanted as much information as possible. Almost all patients in the study wanted to know the *chances of cure* and the *side effects* of their treatments.

Doctors should try their best to give patients adequate information and reverse an increasing reliance on patients' leaflets and videos. Too many doctors have, in the past, adopted the paternalistic view that patients cannot cope with bad news. Patients were seen as 'children' in need of instruction and reassurance rather than experts in their own needs and preferences. Benefits of interventions should be emphasised, and risks and side effects should not be glossed over. Scientific controversies should be mentioned where appropriate. Information given in 'patients' leaflets and videos' should be regularly reviewed and updated. In the UK. and in the European Union, patients' rights are no longer governed by the 'Bolam principle' which states that 'what a reasonable body of physicians decides is acceptable practice'. Patients' rights are now governed by 'what a reasonable patient would wish to know'.

Revalidation for Doctors in the UK

The purpose of *revalidation* is to assure patients and the general public, health care employers and other medical professionals, that doctors on the General Medical Council Register are up to date and fit to practice. The proposed system of revalidation will be based on robust local systems that support high-quality care in organisations and practice settings where that care is delivered. Appraisal and robust clinical governance will remain the key foundation of the process. Revalidation should add value for both patients and doctors and be workable in the current highly pressured and busy environments in which most doctors now work. It is hoped to be a part of a range of measures which ensure high-quality safe health care. It should be simple and streamlined and not place excessive burdens on doctors and their employers.

The *principles* of *revalidation* should include the following:

1. Revalidation must be effective to ensure the General Medical Council (GMC) decisions are carried out properly.
2. Revalidation must be carried out and be based locally and reflect each doctor's actual practice and continuing professional development (CPD).
3. It must be comprehensive and thorough.
4. Revalidation must be fair, non-discriminatory, and consistent.

The attributes to revalidation are that it should be simple, flexible, and supportive to development. It should be capable of reassuring a doctor that he/she can face the end of the revalidation process without surprises.

Benefits to patients by revalidation include protection from poorly performing doctors, promotion of good medical practice, making registration a valid indicator of quality, and increase patients' confidence in doctors on the medical register.

Benefit to doctors: Revalidation may help conscientious doctors show that they are giving good medical care to their patients and encourage them to become even better. It should enable doctors to correct any weaknesses in their practice and improve patients' care and safety in a supportive working environment.

Benefit to employers will be to provide assurance and protection to them on the understanding that the doctors they employ are fit to practice. Employers will have this additional mechanism to identify and deal with poor performances by doctors in partnership with the General Medical Council and other supervisory bodies.

Timetable for revalidation: Subject to the readiness of NHS employers and other health care providers ensuring that they have the local systems in place to support the revalidation of their doctors, the *launch will be in late 2012*. An assessment of readiness will be undertaken in 2012, and it is then when the Secretary of State for Health may commence the relevant legislation in Parliament.

Clinical Risk Management in the NHS, UK

Clinical risk management is a strand of clinical governance, the aim of which is to minimise risk to patients and to encourage good working practices. The ten (10) golden rules of clinical risk management are as follows:

1. Act within your competence.
2. Do no harm to your patients and colleagues.

3. Follow procedures carefully.
4. Report clinical critical incidents including near misses.
5. Give explanations about treatment to patients or their representatives before obtaining consent.
6. Write full, eligible, signed, and dated notes.
7. Maintain patient's confidentiality at all times.
8. Learn from mistakes.
9. Ask if not sure of what you are doing.
10. Always encourage good working practices.

A Flow Chart of Clinical Risk Management:

Identify risk → Analyse and evaluate risk → Control → (Avoid or Prevent) →Accept → Fund → Assure and back to identify risk *or* → Transfer → Monitor → (and back to) Identify risk.

Risk management must have well-rehearsed programmes in place. Human error is inevitable; hence, risk management programmes should endeavour to manage this. In any system, there are three (3) levels at which human error can be managed.

The first level (structure) seeks to decrease the possibility of errors occurring through shaping the behaviour of individuals involved, by careful selection of personnel, by providing appropriate training and continuing medical education (CME), and maintaining good working conditions.

The second level (the process) encourages the detection, absorption, and recovery from the consequences of medical errors.

The third level (the outcome) uses methods appropriate to decrease or minimise the consequences of medical errors.

References

1. Wikipedia, Medical Error, *http://en.wikipedia.org/wiki/ Medical-* error/2011.
2. Harding P. C., Physician Familiarity with the Most Common Misdiagnoses: Implications for Clinical Practice and Continuing Medical Education, *The Intern. J. of Med. Education*, **1**(2), 2010, *www.ispub.com/journal/the-internet-journal/* medical educ
3. Tara Lamont, John Scarpello, National Patient Safety Agency: Combining Stories with Statistics to Minimize Harm, *British Medical Journal*, **339**, 2009,1194-5.
4. Daniel K. Sokol, Can Deceiving Patients Be Morally Acceptable? *British Medical Journal*, **334**, 2007, 984-6.
5. Daniel Sokol, Piers Benn, Medical Ethics. Fresh Insight or Rank Nonsense? *Hospital Doctor*, May 2004, 34, *www.hospital-doctor.net*
6. Jason Ellis, Online Risk Assessment for Revalidation, *MDU Journal*, **19**, 2003, 11, *www.the-mdu.com/GP*
7. Dr Rupert Lee, The 'New' NHS: Modern but Indecipherable? *MDU Journal*, **19**, 2003, 18-19.
8. Susan Mayor, NHS Introduces New Patient Safety Agency, *British Medical Journal*, **322**, 2001, 113.
9. General Medical Council Research, The Role and Responsibilities of Doctors: Protecting Patients and Guiding Doctors, *GMC Booklet*, 2001, *www.gmc-uk.org*
10. Geoff Watts, Coaxing Doctors to Confess, *British Medical Journal*, **321**, 2001, 890.

Chapter 17

Prevention of Medical Errors and Adverse Events

The quest for perfection in the medical profession created sanctions deeply rooted in a philosophy of punishment for poor performance. This produced guilt instead of substantial error reduction. Doctors have been judgemental about their colleagues, and when errors have occurred, their colleagues have felt negative about it and looked down on them, which is inappropriate behaviour. Prevention of medical errors requires attention to systemic causes and the consequences of errors. The multiplicity of mechanisms and causes of medical errors (*internal* and *external*, *individual* and *systemic*) dictates that there cannot be a simple or universal means of reducing errors. Systemic changes are most likely to be successful because they reduce the likelihood of a variety of types of errors at the end-user stage. Creating a safe process requires attention to methods of error reduction at each stage of the system development. This requires responsible individuals at each stage to think through the consequences of their decisions and to reason back from discovered deficiencies and redesign or reorganise the process.

The primary objective of system design for safety is to make it difficult for individuals to err, but it is important to recognise that errors will inevitably occur and so plan for their detection and recovery. Ideally, the system should automatically correct errors when they occur, but if that is impossible, mechanisms should be in place to at least detect errors in time for corrective action. Therefore, in addition to designing the work environment to minimise psychological precursors, designers should provide monitoring functions and building *buffers* and *redundancy*.

Buffers are design features that automatically correct for human or mechanical errors. Redundancy is duplication, triplication, or quadrupling of critical mechanisms and instruments so that failure does not result in loss of function. Another important design feature is designing tasks to minimise errors.

Many health-care systems could be redesigned to significantly reduce the likelihood of errors. Some of the mechanisms that can be used in error prevention are as follows:

a) *Simplification of tasks* to minimise the load on the weakest aspects of cognition, which are short-term memory, planning, and problem solving.

b) *Better ways of identifying negligent behaviour* and the institution of appropriate corrective or disciplinary action. It must be acknowledged that injuries can result from behavioural problems, commonly observed in impaired and incompetent doctors, despite well-designed systems.

c) *Reduction in reliance on memory* by minimising the requirements for human function known to be particularly fallible, such as short-term memory and vigilance. Undertaking system redesign based on well-delineated and understood components of work. Employ more widely checklists, protocols, and computer-based decision aids.

d) *Improved information and its access:* As discussed previously, information should be readily available and be displayed where it is needed, when it is needed, and in a form that permits easy access. Computerisation of medical records would greatly facilitate information access, but even here, power failures and system crashes are known hazards.

e) *Use error proofing* by structuring critical tasks so that errors cannot be made. The use of automatic 'fail-safe' computer safety systems which stop errors being made has proved very helpful and is now widely used. Power of constraints has been exploited. One way to do this is the use of 'forcing functions' which make it impossible to act without meeting a precondition.

f) *Employing standardisation:* Standardising the process or order and delivery of services, whenever possible, can be a most effective means of reducing errors. This process reduces errors by reinforcing the pattern of recognition that humans do well. There are advantages in standardising, like improved efficiency and error reduction in drug administration, where doses and times of administration can be standardised. Information displays and methods for facilitating common practices such as geographic location of equipment and supplies in a health-care unit can also be standardised.

g) *Reversibility* is also very useful in error prevention. Where possible, operations should be easily reversible or difficult to perform when they are not reversible.

h) *Training of medical personnel:* There is a general feeling in the medical profession that *focus* should be on the *training* and *re-accreditation* of doctors in order to improve their standard of practice and morale. Doctors, nurses, and other medical personnel should be trained in the procedures relevant to their specialties and in problem solving, including greater emphasis on safety issues, possible errors, and how to prevent them occurring. Safety issues include understanding the rationale for procedures as well as how errors can occur at various stages; their possible consequences; and instruction in methods for avoidance of errors. Safety practice is as important as effective practice. Doctors need to learn to think of errors primarily as symptoms of system failures.

i) *Clinical critical incident reporting:* Flanagan described critical incident monitoring and reporting way back in 1954 as a result of studies in the aviation psychology programme of the U.S. Air Force during and after the second World War. This description was applied to the practice of Anaesthesia by Cooper and colleagues in 1978 when they defined critical incident as 'an occurrence that could have led, if not discovered or corrected in time, or did lead to an undesirable outcome ranging from increased length of hospital stay, permanent disability, or death'. There are a number of different descriptions of critical incident in use besides this one or the one given in the first chapter of this book.

Anaesthetists in the UK came up with their own description of critical incident as 'an incident which does not necessarily lead to harm but which could or would do so if left to progress'. Adverse events are problems encountered during the process of patient care that cause or had the potential to cause an adverse outcome. Adverse events that do not result in adverse outcomes are classified as *critical incidents*. Any adverse event may have a single adverse outcome, multiple adverse outcomes, or no adverse outcome at all. *Adverse outcomes* are defined as 'patient injury, escalation of care, or operational inefficiencies'.

A critical incident may have an 'alerting event' which acts as early warning, *perceived causes* or *contributory factors* for the event, and *subsequent events*. So it is important to note that several items of information may be useful and are probably essential to be recorded with the incident itself. Contextual information that can be added to the record of an event will enhance subsequent review of the event.

Clinical critical incident reporting by itself does not reduce risk or improve quality. Reporting systems which are used only to collect information are ineffective. They are not used in a systematic way; tend to highlight problems in behaviour rather than clinical risks; and may not be fully embraced and used by the intended staff. They also have a tendency to encourage a fear of incident reporting as a tool of victimisation. Clinical critical incidents need to be discussed in a multidisciplinary forum along with complaints, audits, clinical indicators, and other quality tools. This will encourage their use in highlighting problems with systems and guidelines and allow individuals to learn in a non-threatening environment. Use of monitors to detect changes from normal with speed before injury occurs is now well established in medical practice. In the USA, some states introduced minimum monitoring standards which were to be mandatory by law and enforced by state inspectors. Monitors, however, must be used appropriately and alarms must be set at appropriate levels, and the information they provide must be scanned regularly and interpreted in conjunction with results of the clinical monitoring.

Critical incident data collected centrally should be critically compared and be discussed regularly by the authorities concerned. Analysis of incidents should be the basis of quality improvement plans and give rise to audit and guidelines development. Quality plans should lead to the development of specific incident triggers, which would help focus critical incident reports on those areas of high risk.

Critical Incident Reporting Technique

This has been employed in clinical practice for a long time now as part of the continuous quality improvement (CQI) programme in the National Health Service (NHS) of the UK. Critical incident reporting highlights problems not otherwise covered by case and peer reviews. It complements quality assurance programmes in hospital practice to detect and analyse problems which lead to or may lead to adverse events. Critical incident reporting technique is a form of quality assurance designed to improve patient safety. It is a method of prospectively collecting and analysing data on mishaps or 'near miss' incidents. More information is gathered, and many aspects of the working environment can be continually monitored. Recent problems can be identified, and discussions of events can focus more on prevention than on blame. Voluntary anonymous reporting of incidents encourages a high compliance rate and is essential for reporting human error in particular. It should be remembered that human error is a 'deviation from ideal performance in areas of judgement, technique, and vigilance'.

Critical incident reporting technique is not suitable as a means of quantifying events according to the conventional scientific measurement but continues to be used for several other purposes. *Audit* of work practices facilitates the discovery and correction of factors contributing to the incident and contributes to the teaching and analytical study of how critical incidents evolve. An agreed set of *terms* to describe the incident is essential for national level analysis of critical incidents by computer. This minimises or eliminates duplication or confusion. *Read Clinical Classification,* available and used in the UK, discussed later, has such suitable terms ready for use.

Severity of Adverse Event outcomes and the recording of Incidents

The reporting process of medical errors and adverse events is graded into one of the following categories:

(1) *near miss,* (2) *no injury or sequel,* (3) *injury or sequel,* and (4) *serious sequel or death.*

Cooper and colleagues' definition of critical incident refers to the outcome of the incident, but later, Cooper, Newbower, and Kitz introduced the concept of the substantive negative outcome. The outcome itself cannot be recorded at the time of the incident. However, the importance of a critical incident is related to patient outcome, and so it is essential to be able to include outcomes to the recording of the incident. Classifying outcomes in terms of severity may be enough, but better still, any new diagnosis or condition of the patient so affected need to be recorded as well.

Complication is defined as 'an undesirable condition or diagnosis of a patient which has resulted from medical care'. It may have any grade or severity. It may or may not follow a critical incident. Complication of a critical incident refers to new diagnosis which complicates the previous condition or may refer to problems resulting from post-error medical care. Sometimes it may not be clear if an event is a complication, a critical incident, or both of these. It is almost impossible to separate the two types of terms in a comprehensive set of critical incidents without considering the context in which they have occurred.

Contributing factor is defined as 'a situation of the patient which has led, or could have led to a critical incident or complication in that patient'. The person who labels the event as critical incident should be the person present at the time of the perceived event.

Latent errors in a clinical system may contribute to the occurrence of critical events. Latent errors are *problems* that management can and should address. Incidents caused by latent errors do not tend to recur after their removal, but removal of such errors may be beyond the clinicians' control. Such errors may be those due to drugs' ampoule labelling or faulty equipment not yet replaced. These problems do cause recurrent critical incidents, even though awareness of the problem is increased. Many major disasters ultimately caused by human error would not occur if latent errors known to be in the systems are removed. So it is very important to look for and remove those errors where possible. Where latent errors have been known but not acted upon, they have been the basis for successful litigation against the management of these institutions.

Slip error problem is well known. Making the system safe so that slip errors are less likely to cause a serious incident is probably the best that can be done. Most slip errors reported concern drug administration where dangerous drugs got mixed up and were administered to patients with serious consequences. Specific protocols to specific problems may be effective in reducing the number of incidents of this type.

Read Clinical Classification is a comprehensive *thesaurus* (dictionary) of clinical terms and phrases to which codes (*Read Codes*) are attached. It provides a complete thesaurus of terms, which describe all aspects of clinical medicine. This includes diagnoses, surgical operations, clinical procedures, clinical symptoms, clinical signs, drugs, medical equipments, and the process of health care. The collection of terms was released to the National Health Service (NHS), UK, as a *version 3 of the Read Codes in 1994*. The main advantage of using terms in the Read Code system is that they can be used across the NHS, and they are also computer-coded. They form the basis of standard terminology and can be used as tools for the study of critical incidents. The Read Codes are dynamic and get quarterly updates; they are hierarchical and specifically designed for use in computerised systems. The clinical terms' project contained forty-three medical specialty working groups (SWGs), whose aim was to provide all terms which are deemed to be important to that particular specialty.

In *summary*, each critical incident represents an opportunity for an adverse outcome. A reduction in critical incidents may, in theory, result in a corresponding reduction in adverse outcomes. The critical incident reporting technique elicits the key components of a skill and helps formulate precise teaching objectives in medical education and practice. It replaces introspective, ex-cathedral pontifications by sustained, careful, lengthy, and thoughtful analysis of actual incidents from medical practice. It automatically emphasises incidents of clinical importance, and this method is well suited for examinations that certify minimum professional competence of medical staff.

Clinical guidelines are of two types:

Local clinical guidelines which are locally produced and owned.

National clinical guidelines produced by government agents like the National Institute of Clinical Excellence (NICE) in UK. The Royal colleges participate in setting up national guidelines.

Clinical guidelines have increasingly become part of the current medical practice. They have been proved to change the clinical practice and improve patient-care and health-care outcomes. They help minimise the occurrence of medical errors and adverse events. However, their effectiveness depends on many factors, including the scientific basis or validity of the guidelines and dissemination strategy that promotes compliance.

Guidelines should state explicitly the evidence base from which they are drawn: their author, sponsor, date of production, and date of review or update. If used for culling previous guidelines, they should specify what is being culled. This gives the users the opportunity to draw their own conclusions. Guidelines should be compatible with existing values among the target groups and not be overly controversial. They should not demand too much and cause sudden changes to existing routines. They should be defined precisely with specific advice on actions and decisions in different cases. Some guidelines will inevitably be more effective than others, and none will address all the uncertainties of current clinical practice. They should, therefore, be seen as the only one strategy that can help improve the quality of patient care and minimise the occurrence of medical errors.

Clinical guidelines can also be used in continuing medical education (CME) programmes and to answer specific clinical questions. Valid guidelines can provide an overview of the management of a condition or the use of an intervention. They usually have a broader scope than systemic reviews which tend to focus mainly on an individual problem or intervention. They can provide a more coherent integrated view on how to manage a condition. Guidelines should be used as instruments for self-assessment or peer review and help to learn about gaps in performance and try to bridge them. This is particularly relevant when recommendations have been turned into specific measurable criteria. Doctors and other medical professionals may use guidelines to answer specific clinical questions arising from their day-to-day practice.

The *legal* status of clinical guidelines in the UK is discussed under *litigation*; suffice it to say that doctors are expected to use appropriate clinical discretion, and courts do continue to place the testimony of expert witnesses about what constitutes reasonable practice above the recommendations of prestigious works of reference and certainly above clinical guidelines. Clinical guidelines can be introduced to a court by an expert witness as evidence of accepted and customary standards of health care, but they cannot be introduced as substitute for expert testimony.

Clinical staff induction and training: All new clinical staff, including locum personnel and staff moving to new jobs within their employment, should be given sufficient induction and orientation training to perform the tasks of their posts safely. Induction may be *general*, including clinical risk management, or be *specialty specific*.

The possible dream in the *prevention of medical errors* would be by the establishment of an ideal system the features of which would include the following:

a. Establishment of a strict liability code by which hospitals and related medical institutions bear full responsibility of compensating every injury regardless of fault. This would be met under a *no-fault compensation scheme.*

b. Targeting systems rather than workers and making necessary changes quickly.

c. Driving out fear so that medical errors are freely reported and their causes fully investigated.

d. New approach for training medical staff to work in teams and create multidisciplinary teams to redesign error-prone systems.

e. Stress reduction by the establishment and maintenance of a new focus on working conditions which include targeting long hours, double shifts, poor accommodation, sleep deprivation, and poor irregular meals.

f. Provision of well-organised and resourced continuing education and professional development programmes with revalidation.

g. Full participation in relevant programmes by the pharmaceutical and medical devices industries and other health-care products providers.

h. Participation in the education of patients and the public through improved communication skills.

References

1. Goud et al., Effect of Guideline-based Computerized Decision Support System Decision-making of Multidisciplinary Teams: Cluster Randomized Trial in Cardiac Rehabilitation, *British Medical Journal*, **338**, 2009, b440.

2. Rene Amalberti, et al., Five System Barriers to Achieving Ultrasafe Health Care, *Annals of Intern. Medicine* **142**(9), 2005, 756-64.

3. McBride et al., Preventable Adverse Events in Infants Hospitalized with Bronchiolitis, *Pediatrics*, **116**, 2005, 603-8.

4. Woolf, et al., A String of Mistakes: The Importance of Cascade Analysis, Counting, and Preventing Medical Errors, *Ann. Fam. Med.*, **2**, 2004, 317-19.
5. Peter Walsh, Outlines of How Action Against Medical Accidents (AvMA) Will Get Patients and Public Involved in Patient Safety and Clinical Governance Work, *GMC News*, 27 December 2004.
6. Dominic Bell, Avoiding Adverse Outcomes When Faced with 'Difficult' Ventilation, *Anaesthesia*, **58**, 2003, 945-50.
7. Prof. Chris Bulstrode, On Course to Change the Face of Training, *Hospital Doctor* (UK), February 1999, 38.
8. Dr P. Verow, Occupational Doctor Can Help, *Hospital Doctor* (UK), April 1999, 14.
9. Martin Hutchinson, Revalidation a Lash Too Far for Doctors? *Hospital Doctor* (UK), February 1999, 2-3.
10. Martin Hutchinson, *Hospital Doctor* (UK) February 1999, 34.
11. Dr Edwin Borman, Revalidation the Way Forward, *Hospital Doctor* (UK), February 1999, 40.
12. Gene Feder, Martin Eccles, et al., Use of Guidelines by Clinicians, *British Medical Journal*, **318**, 1999, 730.
13. Department of Health, Guidance in Implementing Clinical Governance in the NHS, *HS Circular* 1999/065.
14. D. Irvine, The Performance of Doctors: the New Professionalism, *The Lancet*, 1999, 1174-7.
15. Graham Buckley, Revalidation Is the Answer, *British Medical Journal*, **319**, 1999, 1145-6.
16. Jenis Smy, What Does Clinical Governance Mean? *Hospital Doctor* (UK), February 1999, 30.
17. John Parboosingh, Revalidation for Doctors, *British Medical Journal*, **317**, 1998, 1094-5.
18. Philip Bashook, J. Parboosingh, Recertification and Maintenance of Competence, *British Medical Journal*, **316**, 1998, 545-8.
19. D. Seedhouse, Should Mandatory Ethics Programme Be Established for All Doctors? *Hospital Doctor* (UK), November 1998, 54.
20. Tessa Richards, Continuing Medical Education, *British Medical Journal*, **316**, 1998, 246.
21. Sir Donald Irvine, Performance of Doctors: Maintaining Good Practice; Protecting Patients from Poor Performance, *British Medical Journal*, **314**, 1997, 1613-15.

22. Sir Donald Irvine, The Performance of Doctors: Professionalism and Self-regulation in a Changing World, *British Medical Journal*, **314**, 1997, 1540-2.

23. Gabriel Scally, Tackling Deficient Doctors, *British Medical Journal*, **314**, 1997, 1568.

24. J. Santell, Professional Organizations in Other Countries to Combat Medical Negligence, *British Medical Journal*, **315**, 1997, 970.

25. Julia von Onciul, Stress at Work, *British Medical Journal*, **313**, 1996, 745-7.

26. Rebecca Voelker, Treat Systems, Not Errors; Experts Say, *Journal of the American Medical Association*, **276**(19), 1996, 1537-8.

27. T. G. Short, A. O'Regan, et al., Improvements in Anaesthetic Care Resulting from a Critical Incident Reporting Programme, *Anaesthesia*, **51**, 1996, 615-21.

28. Prof. Lucian Leape, Error in Medicine, *Journal of the American Medical Association*, **272**(23), 1994, 1851-7.

29. I. Banks, R. M. Tackley, A Standard Set of Terms for Critical Incident Recording, *Brit. J. Anaesthesia*, **73**, 1994, 703-8.

30. Donaldson L.J, Doctors with Problems in a National Health Service Workforce, *British Medical Journal*, **308**, 1994, 1277-82.

31. T. Short, A. O'Regan, et al., Critical Incident Reporting in Anaesthetic Department: Quality Assurance Programme, *Anaesthesia*, **47**, 1992, 3-7.

32. Prof. Lucian Leape, Troyen A. Brennan, et al., The Nature of Adverse Events and Negligence in Hospitalized Patients, *The New Engl. J. Med.*, **324**(26), 1991, 377-84.

33. R. J. Asher, Critical Questions: Critical Incidents: Critical Answers, *The Lancet*, 1988, 1373-4.

34. A. Simanowitz, Standards, Attitudes and Accountability in the Medical Profession, *The Lancet*, 1985, 546-7.

35. R. Newbower, R.J. Kitz, An Analysis of Major Errors and Equipment Failures in Anesthesia Management: Considerations for Prevention and Detection, *Anesthesiology*, **60**, 1984, 34-42.

36. N. McIntyre and K. Popper, The Critical Attitude in Medicine: Need for New Ethics, *British Medical Journal*, **287**, 1983, 1919-23.

Chapter 18

Medical Devices, Equipments, and Medical Errors

A *medical device is defined* as 'any health care product, excluding drugs, which is used for a patient in the diagnosis, treatment, prevention or alleviation of illness or injury'. So a medical device could be a sophisticated CT scanner or it might equally be a hip joint prosthesis or a bandage. There is an increasing use of very sophisticated devices in the medical profession worldwide. Some devices will be easier to use safely than others, but all of them will have to be adequately understood by end users, mainly through proper training and supervision, if medical errors and adverse medical incidents are to be minimised or avoided altogether. The language used in end-user instruction manuals needs to be adequately understood by them if confusion and user paralysis is to be avoided. Computer literacy is now a must for all as modern medical equipment operations are computer-based.

Different medical equipments give warnings in different ways. They can be *audio*, *visual displays*, or a combination of these two. Some warnings may be false alarms, but manufacturers have worked hard to minimise and eventually eliminate such false responses in modern machines and equipments. All warnings from them must be attended to urgently. Knowledge and experience with the device being used should help the user make quick, sensible, and safe decisions as regards the significance of the warnings and take the appropriate action. Remember, warnings can result either from a *device fault* or from an *operator error*.

Training doctors in the use of new medical equipments should be obligatory and be a part of continuing medical education. Doctors should not come across new equipments at the workplace and depend on the user manuals for safe and efficient use on their patients. Old and more familiar equipments should be handy as back-up in these situations. In the NHS, with the establishment of a multitude of trusts, suppliers of medical equipments do differ from trust to trust, delivering different models and types of products. As medical personnel move from one NHS trust to another in search of better environment or for further training and future promotion, the problem of 'equipment diversity' needs urgent evaluation although one may argue that this may be one of the incentives for staff to make a move and learn more.

The Medical Devices Agency (UK) is a government agency in the Department of Health and deals with the safety of medical devices and monitors safety standards in their manufacture if made here in the UK. It is responsible for the safety, quality, and effectiveness of all medical devices used in the NHS trusts and associated health-care providers. It inspects and registers manufacturers of medical devices. The agency tests devices and publishes a wide range of bulletins, product reports, and guidelines aimed at the manufacturers and end users of devices. It is also involved in developing standards across the world and gives technical advice to the Department of Health, community and hospital NHS trusts, and many other health service organisations.

The agency has played a role in the establishment of a European Union single organisation to deliver on a series of medical devices directives which apply throughout the member states and in the European Free Trade Association (EFTA). Since 14 June 1998, all medical devices marketed in the European Union (EU) have to comply with the Medical Devices Directive 93/42/EEC. If devices have faults or malfunction, the agency coordinates investigations into their causes and helps to prevent them happening again. It issues warnings to users of any item proved to be or suspected to be unsafe. However, the agency cannot be there to safeguard patients and medical staff when devices are in day-to-day use.

The medical staff have to fulfil this role as it is their responsibility to protect patients and to act as eyes and ears for the agency. The agency advises medical staff to be prepared to be questioned about the way they handle devices in their use and encourages them to develop an acute awareness of the capability and limitations of these devices. Users should also be adequately knowledgeable as regards the state of repair and service history of the devices in their regular use.

When equipments are in use, the importance of reading instructions carefully, understanding them, and acting upon them even if one uses that particular equipment regularly cannot be overemphasised. Medical physics technicians, electro-medical engineers, radiation protection officers, sterile service managers, and health and safety officers are some of the medical personnel who should be useful trainers of other staff members as they are involved in the safe use and maintenance of medical devices.

The CE Mark

The CE mark on medical devices demonstrates that the device conforms with one of the two directives passed by the Council of Ministers of the European Union. The two directives require manufacturers who wish to sell devices within the European Union to submit their devices to a conformity assessment procedure in order to confirm that a device has been manufactured within the terms of a 'quality system', either through a comprehensive BS/ EN/ ISO 900-type system or other systems like type testing and sample analysis.

The *first* directive, the *Active Implantable Medical Devices Directive* which applies to devices such as pacemakers and cochlear implants, was introduced in the UK in January 1993 and implemented in January 1995. Devices of this type manufactured or sold within the European Union must carry a CE mark.

The *second* directive, *the Medical Devices Directive,* was introduced in the UK on 1 January 1995 and applies to the remainder of medical devices.

These directives stipulate that each member state of the EU must have a 'two-tier regulatory authority', which in turn designates and monitors independent certification organisations called *notified bodies (NBs)*. The CE mark shows that the device or service offered meets the essential requirements of the relevant directive. It means that the manufacturer can claim that the product satisfies the requirements essential for it to be considered but not guaranteed safe and fit for its intended purpose. Before applying the CE marking to a product or its packaging, a manufacturer must go through one or more conformity assessment procedures to confirm that the design and production of the product meet all relevant requirements laid down in the directive. The CE mark also means that the product can be freely marketed anywhere in the EU without further control. The stringency of these procedures depends on which directive applies and on the classification of the medical product concerned.

Devices without the CE marking are of two types: devices covered by the transitional arrangements laid down in each directive and devices intended for special purposes.

British Standards Institute has a 'Kite' mark which appears on many different types of products. The British Standards prefix followed by four (4) digits, BS 5750, is the National Standards for quality systems. It is general in scope and applies to every kind of industry in the UK. It indicates that the contractor has the quality system in place to meet the needs of the customer and end user. The 'Crown and Tick' symbol was awarded to organisations which applied successfully for registration under the British National Standard BS 5750. Most British National Standards are far more specific. BS 4272 applies solely to anaesthetics and analgesia-administering machines. BS 2463 applies to intravenous administration (infusion) sets. BS 3221 applies to medicine measures.

There are other *international standards* which are set and supervised by such organisations as the European Committee for Standardization (CEN) and the European Committee for Electro-technical Standardization (CENELEC), both based in Brussels, the International Organization for Standardization (ISO), and the International Electro-technical Commission (IEC). There is commonality of standards between these organisations which share knowledge and expertise, thereby reducing wasteful duplication between member states of the EU. Many British Standards have equivalents internationally. BS 5750 series are equivalent to EN 2900 and ISO 9000 series.

A well-researched and prepared standard helps manufacturers develop products which are safe, effective, and appropriate to their application. Standards help those buying medical devices identify products appropriate to their needs. They reassure medical personnel that the industry is committed to providing better and safer products. This boosts confidence in the products' effectiveness and safety. Most standards, however, have been voluntary, and manufacturers have been under no legal obligation to conform.

Medical Devices and Professional Accountability

Professional accountability calls for each individual to continuously question his/her own practice and not to take things for granted. Routines should not obscure priorities. Safety demands continuous and committed effort from health care professionals to meet their obligations. When adverse incidents occur, the primary contact in the UK is the *adverse incident centre (AIC)*. The purpose of this reporting procedure is to facilitate centrally coordinated action to safeguard patients and staff. This may take the form of a warning circular or a product recall. This process has led to improved design, improved manufacturing processes, better labelling, and clearer instructions to the end users. The AIC sends out hazard warnings and safety notices to the appropriate medical institutions, and these instructions are product specific. Hazard warnings are used in the most serious cases when either a patient's life has been put at risk or when staff safety has been compromised. Immediate action should follow when a hazard warning is received. Safety notices are issued when it is clear that a potential safety problem exists in a device or in a system that it is a part of. They call for action to avoid risk, often involving alerting the staff or altering procedures either for use or maintenance of the equipment. Safety notices are also used to report warnings on long-standing problems or to follow up manufacturers' field modifications, ensuring that end users are aware and have the necessary modifications completed.

Basic principles to follow when a *medical equipment in use fails* include the following:

1. Protect the patient and make things safe for all involved.
2. Keep the equipment or device involved in the incident, including packaging and relevant instructions, for examination by the appropriate personnel.
3. For a machine, leave all switches and controls as they were at the time of the incident unless it is unsafe to do so, say where electrical short circuits may be involved.
4. Decontaminate the equipment before submitting it for examination as specified in HSG (93).26/U.K. The unit safety officer is usually responsible for carrying out this procedure.
5. Do not surrender the equipment to the manufacturer or allow interference with any part of it before it is examined by the

designated authority in the local procedure and by the Medical Devices Agency staff, if appropriate.

6. If the item is part of a batch, check the remaining stock and assess if the defect has anything to do with storage, expiry date, or poor handling. If in doubt, take the rest of the batch out of circulation as a safety measure.

7. Misuse of equipment or mistakes made by the user for any reason should be identified and appropriate action taken to avoid a repeat. Lessons should be learnt through the actions taken through the unit critical incident reporting and management systems.

8. There should be easy access to emergency services. The Medical Devices Agency, through its adverse incident centre (AIC), provides these contact services:

Tel.: 020 71 972 8080; *Fax*: 020 71 972 8109, Web site: *www. medical-services.gov.uk*

Other countries have similar *protocols* for the use and maintenance of medical equipments by professionals in an effort to eliminate or minimise the occurrence of errors and adverse incidents.

Doctors in *Norway* are obliged by law to submit reports of injuries and risks of injury arising from the use of medical equipments and drugs to central authorities. Most hospitals in Norway have their own rules requiring health care providers to report all incidents resulting in injury or risk of injury to the appropriate authorities.

In the US, the Safe Medical Devices Act (SMDA) of 1990 mandated the reporting of complications related to the use of medical devices to the United States Food and Drug Administration. This act empowered the Food and Drug Administration to require many health-care facilities to investigate, document, and report serious events related to all types of medical devices, some of which had to be tracked from receipt, through patient use, to disposal. The act placed legal responsibility on health care practitioners to assess and report malfunctioning medical equipments. Lack of compliance would carry civil and criminal penalties, affect liability and risk management, and influence the accreditation of physicians.

With the issue and implementation of Medical Devices Directives in the EU, there has been an attempt to streamline arrangements for reporting and acting on adverse incidents involving medical devices. Under the medical device vigilance system, manufacturers are required by law to report serious incidents involving their devices, recall or withdraw of devices, to the relevant competent authority, e.g. the Medical Devices Agency in the UK. Information collected and evaluated by a *member state* of the *EU* may be made available to the other member states. This system was aimed at allowing information to be shared across Europe, and any problems reported were to be addressed quickly and systematically.

References

1. Dr Susanne Ludgate, Medical Equipment Safety: Not Left to Its Own Devices, *MDU Journal*, **19**, 2003, 14-15, *www.medical-devices. gov.uk*
2. J. Amoore, P. Ingram, Medical Devices: Learning from Adverse Incidents, *British Medical Journal*, 325(272) (ED), 2005, 905(L).
3. *EU Council Directive* 93/42/EEC, June 1993.
4. *Official Journal* L 169, July 1993, 0001-43.

Chapter 19

Medical Errors in Prescribing and Dispensing of Drugs

Prescribing and drug administration errors and their prevention are continuously being addressed by drug companies and medical personnel as end users. Prescribing and administering drugs is a complex process as it involves several people, usually the one prescribing, the pharmacist, nurses, and other health care staff. Some of those administering drugs may be relatives of patients and have minimal or no knowledge of the drugs they administer. It is not surprising, therefore, that drug errors do occur.

A study carried out way back in 1993 by B. S. Dean, E. L. Allan, et al. compared medication errors in an *American* and a *British hospital*. Following is the summary of their study and findings, and I quote:

Medication errors in a hospital in the U.S. and a hospital in the U.K. were compared. The U.S. hospital was studied in August 1993 and the U.K. hospital was studied in May and June 1993. The U.S. hospital had a typical unit drug distribution system, and the U.K. hospital had the ward-based system commonly used in the U.K. in which a Pharmacist makes several visits daily to Wards to review patients' medication charts. The medication chart is used by the physician to order drugs and obviates the need for transcription of orders.

A distinguished observation-technique was used to determine frequencies and types of medical errors. Medication errors were identified retrospectively in the U.S. hospital by comparing the observer's notes with the original drug orders made in the patient's chart by the physician.

In the U.K. hospital, observation of errors took place concurrently; as doses were administered, they were compared with the orders on the medication charts. In the U.S. and the U.K. hospitals, 919 and 2756 opportunities for error were observed respectively. The medication error rate in the U.S. hospital was 6.9 per cent, significantly higher than the 3.0 per cent rate observed in the U.K. hospital;

Omitted doses and incorrect doses were the most common types of errors in the U.K. hospital. Incorrect doses and un-ordered doses were the most common types of errors in the U.S. hospital. An American hospital with a unit dose distribution system had a significantly higher medication error rate than a British hospital with a ward-based supply system.

In a survey done in Boston, USA, published in *Journal of the American Medical Association*, **274,** 1995, 29-34 by D. W. Bates et al., prescribing and drug administration errors accounted for 25 per cent of all drug-related adverse events which occurred in 6.5 per cent of patients admitted into hospital. Near misses accounted for 5.5 per cent of these patients.

Contributory factors in the occurrence of errors in prescribing and administration of drugs include failure to understand and follow instructions, patients having similar names; use of non-approved or abbreviated names, use of unclear dosage units, transcription prescribing errors, confused dosage for different routes of drug administration, over-dosage, wrong intervals or periods between administration of drugs, and use of wrong equipments to administer drugs.

Prevention of Drug Prescription and Administration Errors

This involves proper training of medical personnel, legible handwriting, proper communication between staff and patients, proper labelling of drugs, proper instructions in the use and routes of administration of drugs, using the right equipment, carefully programming drug-delivery equipments, paying particular attention to drug allergies, known side effects, and drug interactions, investigating reported problems by patients, and getting a full history of the patient's other medications. Regular and thorough evaluation of the ever-changing clinical condition of a patient should minimise the occurrence of drug-related adverse events in clinical practice.

The use of computers may obviate some of these problems, but computers can cause problems of their own. Transfer of patients' information to the computer must be thorough and complete and must be updated regularly especially with regard to repeat prescriptions and after every referral to specialists or a hospital admission. Patients, on discharge from the hospital, should have 'discharge medicine lists' which show the indication for each medicine and the intended period of treatment. Doctors should review patients on repeat prescriptions regularly to ensure that such medicine is still necessary, effective, well-tolerated, and appropriate in the context of other medications being taken. Drugs should be linked with diagnoses so that the original reason for the prescription can be ascertained. Overuse, underuse, review dates, sensitivities and allergies, and interactions should be programmed under warnings.

Names and formulations of drugs can be a source of confusion. Pharmacists with access to patients' records on the computer may detect these types of errors. Specialist drugs should be dispensed by senior personnel and their administration be supervised or monitored by senior staff, if appropriate. Drug-dosage errors tend to occur more often in children, the elderly, and the critically ill patients. They also occur quite often when small doses are to be calculated and administered. An example is the administration of *insulin* in diabetic patients. Using tables and other specific instructions may be helpful, but when in doubt, drugs should not be administered to a patient under any circumstances.

In conclusion, drug-related errors and adverse events can occur at all stages of prescribing, dispensing, and administration of drugs. Clear prescriptions and taking care over details of dosage, route of administration, frequency of administration, and period of administration are essential in the endeavour to prevent errors. The correct drug, concentration, the right form of the drug, the state of drug solution, the expiry date, all must be checked very carefully before the drug is administered to a patient. Routes of administration should be confirmed and sites of parenteral administration should be inspected regularly looking for leaks, blockages, swellings, colour changes to the skin, painful sites, and loss of sensation or loss of movement, where limbs have been used. The pharmaceutical industry should act to reduce errors in drug administration by proper, well-considered labelling of drug ampoules, proper labelling of bags of solutions, and providing proper instructions on drug packaging. Strict and enforceable use of colour codes which are understood and accepted by end users should be promoted although this in itself cannot rule out human error.

Recent cases related to Drug Prescription and Administration Errors

Case 1. *Birth drug kills mum*: A mum of two died after being given a labour-inducing drug sixteen (16) times the recommended dose. She was given Misoprostol 800 mcg instead of the recommended 50 mcg. This happened at St. George's Hospital, Tooting, South London UK (taken from *Daily Mirror*, Friday, 3 June 2011: 28).

Case 2. *Fatal dose, nurse banned*: An 'overworked' nurse who accidentally killed a grandmother with a lethal insulin dose was suspended for a year. The diabetic patient was given 3.6 ml dose instead of 0.36 ml dose of insulin. This happened at Mount Surgery, Pontypool, Gwent, Wales, UK (taken from *Daily Mirror*, Friday, 3 June 2011: 28).

Case 3. *An epidural anaesthetic drug* (in an infusion bag) was administered to a woman in labour in her *arm* instead of into her (*lumbar*) *spine* at Great Western Hospital, Swindon, and Marlborough NHS Trust, UK, with fatal consequences. This happened in May 2004. (taken from *Daily Mail*, 19 June 2006).

Case 4. *A newly qualified pharmacist* and a pre-registration pharmacist were charged with manslaughter after making an error with the amount of *chloroform* they added to a preparation of *peppermint water* which led to the death of a three-year-old baby. This happened in 1998 here in the UK.

References

1. Tom Jefferson et al., Ensuring Safe and Effective Drugs: Who Can Do What It Takes? *British Medical Journal*, **342**, 2011, 148-51.

2. Tom Jefferson et al., *British Medical Journal*, **342**, 2011, 183.

3. M. A. Ghaleb, N. Barber, et al., The Incidence and Nature of Prescribing and Medication Administration on Errors in Paediatric In-patients, *Arch. Dis. Child.*, 2010: (2010), adc.2009.15645vl.

4. McDowell et al., Where Errors Occur in the Preparation of Intravenous Medicines: A Systematic Review and Bayesian Analysis, *Postgrad. Med. J.*, **86**, 2010, 734-8.

5. Roberts et al., Impact of Health Information Technology on Detection of Potential Adverse Drug Events at the Ordering Stage, *Am. J. Health Syst. Pharm.*, **67**, 2010, 1838-46.

6. Magrabi et al., An Analysis of Computer-related Patient Safety Incidents to Inform the Development of a Classification, *J. Am. Med. Inform Assoc.* **17**, 2010, 663-70.

7. Condren et al., Prescribing Errors in a Pediatric Clinic: Impact of a Standard Medication Chart on Prescribing Errors Before and After Audit, *Qual. Safe Health Care*, **18**, 2009, 478-85.

8. van Doormaal et al., The Influence that Electronic Prescribing Has on Medication Errors and Preventable Adverse Drug Errors, *J. Am. Med. Inform. Assoc.*, **16**, 2009, 816-25.

9. Singh et al., Prescription Errors and Outcomes Related to Inconsistent Information Transmitted Through Computerized Order Entry, *Arch. Intern. Med.*, **169**, 2009, 982-9.

10. vanDoormaal et al., Medication Errors: The Impact of Prescribing and Transcribing Errors on Preventable Harm in Hospitalized Patients, *Qual. Safe Health Care*, **18**, 2009, 22-27.

11. Conroy and Carroll, Prescribing in Children: Education and Practice, **94**, 2009, 55-9.

12. Kopel et al., Identifying and Quantifying Medication Errors: Evaluation of Rapidly Discontinued Medication Orders Submitted to a Computerized Physician Order Entry System, *J. Am. Med. Inform. Assoc.*, **15**, 2008, 461-5.

13. Jha et al., Can Surveillance Systems Identify and Avert Adverse Drug Events? *J. Am. Med. Inform. Assoc.* **17**, 2008, 286-90.

14. Sari et al., Incidence, Preventability and Consequences of Adverse Events in Elderly, *J. Age-Aging*, **37**, 2008, 265-9.

15. J. H. Simpson, Grant J., How Can We Reduce Medication Errors in the Neonatal Intensive Care Unit? *B. J. Intensive Care* (Spring Issue) 2006, 19-21.

16. Dean B. Schachter, M. Vincent et al., Causes of Prescribing Errors in Hospital Patients: a Prospective Study, *The Lancet*, **359**, 2002, 1373-8.

17. Maxwell et al., Prescriptions: Undergraduate Education, *British Medical Journal*, **324**, 2002, 930.

18. Jeremy Lawrence, Patients at Risk from Hospital Drug Errors, *The Independent*, 5 December 2002.

19. Kanshal R., Bates. D. W., et al., Medication Errors and Adverse Drug events in Paediatric Inpatients, *Journal of the American Medical Association*, **285**, 2001, 2114-20.

20. T. Lesar, L. Briceland, et al., Factors Related to Errors in Medication Prescribing, *Journal of the American Medical Association*, **277**, 1997, 312-17.
21. A. G. Zermansky, Who Controls Repeats? *Br. J. Gen. Practice*, **46**, 1996, 643-7.
22. C. M. Harris, R. Dajda, The Scale of Repeat Prescribing, *Br. J. Gen. Practice*, **46**, 1996, 649-53.
23. D. Bates; D. Cullen, et al., Incidence of Adverse Drug Events and Potential Drug Events: Implications for Prevention, *Journal of the American Medical Association*, **274**, 1995, 29-34.
24. B.S. Dean, E. Allan, et al., Comparison of Medical Errors in an American and a British Hospital, *American Journal of Health-System Pharmacy*, **52**(22), 1995, 2543-9.
25. J. Gladstone, Drug Administration Errors: a Study into the Factors Underlying the Occurrence and Reporting of Drug Errors in a District General Hospital, *J. Adv. Nursing*, **22**, 1995, 628-37.
26. R. E. Ferner, Is There a Cure for Drug Errors? *Journal of the American Medical Association*, **311**, 1995, 463-4.
27. J. K. Aronson, Routes of Drug Administration: Intramuscular Injection, *Prescribers' Journal* (UK), **35**, 1995, 32-6.
28. D. H. Cousins, D. R. Upton, et al., Reducing the Risks of Chemotherapy Errors, *Hospital Pharmacist* (UK), **5**, 1995, 117-20.
29. G. Hill, The KCL killer, *J. Med. Defence Union* (UK), **6**, 1990, 10-11.
30. S. N. Fine, R. M. Eisdorfer, et al., *Losec or Lasix? The New Engl. J. Med.*, **322**, 1990, 1674.

Conclusion

In conclusion, one should look at some of the areas in training doctors and their practice of medicine where changes need to be made in order to minimise the occurrence of medical errors and the severity of adverse events whatever their causes. The emphasis in current medical training centres on diagnosis, treatment, and prevention of potentially dangerous medical conditions. Doctors' training in dealing with the *aftermath of crises* has been patchy and non-intensive. The aftermath has often been handled haphazardly and in an insensitive manner with adverse consequences for the patient, relatives, and medical staff. Drawing up a contingency plan to minimise the trauma and stress which inevitably results, when the unexpected disaster occurs, is now a must for each and every specialty in medical practice.

In reading this book, one will have already begun the preparation for prevention of medical errors and, when the inevitable occurs, to properly manage the aftermath. Some doctors might have faced such situations before and have regrets about the manner in which they handled these unfortunate events in their careers. Some aspects of their experience might have been different if better training and good information sources were available to them at the time.

As this book goes into libraries, it may contain information that is out of date due to improvements resulting from the constant reviews and advances in medical science and medical practice. As Professor Eden said, 'All high risk specialties are facing a twin challenge. Technical and medical advances mean more and more can be attempted but the expectation of the public is of total care for every illness, with decreasing tolerance of any failure to occur'. High expectations often lead to anger and a search for reprisal. Professor Eden called for a change in the culture of distrust and the equation of any complication or poor outcomes with negligence.

References

1. General Medical Council, Good Medical Practice: Duties of a Doctor, 2010, *www.gmc-uk.org/guide/good* medical practice
2. General Medical Council, Good Medical Practice: Raising Concerns About Patient Safety, 2010, *www.gmc-uk.org/guide/good* medical practice

Glossary

About the Author
Dr David Daniel Falijala Waluube

Dr David Waluube is a sixty-seven-year-old Anaesthetist who worked in the National Health Service (NHS), UK, for about thirty years before retiring in December 2008. He is married and has grown-up children one of whom is a manager in the NHS. David was born in Uganda where he studied at Busoga College Mwiri, Kings College Buddo, before going to the East African University, Makerere Medical School, in 1965. At Makerere University, David was a good debator and a keen researcher in Paediatrics for which work he was awarded prizes. He was Editor of Makerere Medical Students' Journal for three years.

David is well-travelled and worked in maternal and child health services of Nairobi City Council, Kenya, for eight years and the Ministry of Health, British Guyana, as a Surgeon and General Practitioner for over a year, before joining the NHS in 1979 at Northampton District General Hospital. He trained at The Royal Liverpool University Hospital and had a stint in Obstetric anaesthesia at St. Thomas Hospital, London. He worked in many subspecialties of Anaesthesia except for Neuro and Cardiothoracic. His last post was of an Associate Specialist in Anaesthesia at the William Harvey Hospital, Ashford, Kent.

Dr Waluube contributed to debates and discussions on improving junior doctors working conditions, especially conditions for locum doctors who were regularly and habitually accused of being the source of many medical errors in the NHS. He produced a booklet for patients on "pain relief in labour and delivery" as a "work for hire" while working at the William Harvey Hospital. His next publication is a Medical Abbreviations Dictionary.

David has been engaged in sending medical materials and medical equipments to Uganda where he visits regularly and gives training and lectures to doctors and medical assistants. Medical errors may be getting less common in developed countries than previously reported but when they occur, many are dramatic, drastic, and do involve a lot of intensive interventions. In developing countries, such occurrences always lead to catastrophic consequences for the patient.

Dr Waluube offers this book as a small but important contribution to the understanding of the underlying causes of medical errors and adverse events, how to avoid them and be prepared to deal with their aftermath promptly and professionally when they occur. The book is relevant and highly recommended to medical students, a privilege their peers never had as undergraduates.

Dr David. D. F. Waluube: M.B,Ch.B (East Africa); D.A; MRCA (London).
E-mail: dwaluube@hotmail.co.uk